The New Anti-Inflammatory Diet Cookbook for Beginners

THE ESSENTIAL GUIDE TO WELL-BEING. EASY AND DELICIOUS RECIPES TO HEAL THE IMMUNE SYSTEM AND REDUCE INFLAMMATION, WITH 30 DAYS MEAL PLAN

Nancy Vassallo

CONTENTS

FOREWORD:

Thank you for purchasing this book. The Anti-Inflammatory Diet is more than just a fad – it's a scientifically backed approach to nutrition that can help alleviate a wide range of health problems, from joint pain to digestive issues to fatigue. And with the help of renowned nutritionist and industry expert Nancy Vassallo, you can learn how to adopt this powerful way of eating and start feeling better in no time.

In this book, Nancy Vassallo provides a comprehensive anti-inflammatory diet guide, covering everything from the basics of inflammation to the specific foods and nutrients that can help fight it. You'll learn about the underlying causes of inflammation, such as stress, poor sleep, and environmental toxins, and how certain foods can exacerbate or ease these symptoms.

But the real power of this book lies in her practical advice and advice. Vassallo provides clear, easy-to-follow instructions on how to adopt an anti-inflammatory diet, including a 30-day meal plan.

But what sets this book apart is her focus on personalization. Vassallo understands that everyone's body is different and that there is no one-size-fits-all approach to nutrition. Whether you're dealing with chronic pain, digestive issues, or just general fatigue, this book has the tools and knowledge you need to start feeling better.

And the benefits of an anti-inflammatory diet go far beyond just physical health. Studies have shown that a diet rich in anti-inflammatory foods can also improve mental health by reducing symptoms of anxiety and depression. So not only will you feel better physically, but you will also take care of your mental and emotional well-being.

But we know that changing your diet can be a daunting task, especially if you've tried other fad diets with no success. That's why this book is designed to be accessible and supportive, providing you with the information and guidance you need to make lasting changes in your eating habits.

With its comprehensive approach, tailored advice and practical advice, it is the perfect guide for anyone who wants to improve their health and well-being through the power of nutrition.

CHAPTER 1

INTRODUCTION

When combating inflammation, you know you are in a hard battle. There is so much going on in your body and mind that it is frequently overwhelming and tiring.

After all, weariness is a sign of inflammation for a reason! You will find different strategies and approaches throughout this book and your research to help you adopt an anti-inflammatory lifestyle and live a healthy life, but even this might be daunting.

Creating an action plan is one of the most vital pieces of advice you may ever get in this struggle. It implies that you must do more than declare your intention to prioritize your health and reduce the burden of chronic inflammation on your life. It involves considering how you will integrate it into your life. It involves producing a statement that is actionable and specific.

Consider addressing your water use as one example. You cannot just resolve to drink more water each day. You should select how much and how you will increase your daily water intake.

Use this basic water example to construct a realistic and executable strategy by following the steps below: Identify your present activities and be sincere!

Regarding the water illustration, how much water do you currently consume?

Do not attempt to be "excellent" throughout your observation; instead, be genuine. How much do you spend on average every day? Being truthful allows you to establish a foundation upon which to grow.

Cheating and attempting to do more than normal during this period will set you up for failure. Instead, perform your customary actions and go from there.

What do you wish to achieve that is feasible? It expresses the particular aspect you wish to enhance. You do not say here, 'drink more water.'

You state, "Increase the quantity of water I consume daily from five to eight cups." Or, "Drink a minimum of nine glasses of water daily."

Be clear and attainable while setting your objective. How will you attain this objective? Will you set the alarm to remind you to drink a couple of cups of water?

Or do you want a fresh bottle you can fill with your regular water intake and drink from throughout the day, ensuring that it is empty before you go to bed?

It would help if you defined how you will monitor your progress toward your objective and what tools you will employ to get it. It may vary when you begin working towards your objective, but the notion is particular to what you intend to attempt.

For instance, if you find it impractical to carry a large water bottle about all day, you may select a smaller bottle that you need to replace three times during the day and set the alarm to remind you to finish and replenish during the day.

It indicates that you modify your strategy's "how" component but not the objective. Instead, focus on the little, attainable steps you may take to achieve your greater health objectives. Apply this formula to the dietary modifications you intend to make while on the anti-inflammatory diet.

Consider how you approach your weekly fruit and vegetable consumption and fish consumption.

Discuss how you want to eliminate sweets and saturated fats, manage exceptional events, and the inevitable temptations that will arise.

Please do not overwhelm yourself with a million action plans; instead, choose a few to focus on and keep adding to them as you create new anti-inflammatory behaviors. Remember that your life and relationship with food are at stake.

Because we are all unique, your body may react differently to food than someone else's. It means your strategy may differ from someone else's, which is okay!

Choose a modification you wish to make, then include it in your unique plan. Move on to your steps after discovering a distinction and 'how' that works for your life and requirements.

Listed below are various modifications that will assist you in adopting an anti-inflammatory diet. Some are "Do," and others are "Do not."

What exactly is It?

The anti-inflammatory diet is not just for weight loss. However, weight loss is a possible side effect. It takes more than three weeks to eliminate present inflammation from the body.

There is no false shortcut to wellness. It presents a unique approach to living: a way of life that includes all the nutrients, minerals, calories, and proteins needed to live a healthy and happy existence.

The anti-inflammatory diet will improve your general health by supplying your body with the nutrients and inflammation-fighting substances it needs to recover and maintain equilibrium.

You will begin to experience physical and mental changes. You will have a revitalized sense of vitality. Your skin will radiate a distinct healthy shine.

Your body will function properly, generate new healthy cells, and decrease the inflammation inside your system.

One must comprehend to adhere to the anti-inflammatory diet and realize its health benefits.

Principal Advantages of Anti-Inflammatory Diet:

According to studies, an anti-inflammatory diet may alleviate the symptoms of various diseases.

Atherosclerosis is the accumulation of plaque in the arteries and is prevalent among the elderly. The researchers discovered a correlation between subclinical atherosclerosis and mortality from heart disease; adhering to an anti-inflammatory diet can help reduce particular inflammatory markers in type 2 diabetes patients.

People with type 2 diabetes who strictly adhere to the suggested Mediterranean diet had fewer inflammation symptoms than those who do not follow any anti-inflammatory diet.

Significant parallels exist between the **Mediterranean diet** and an anti-inflammatory diet. The Mediterranean diet entails selecting and cooking protein-rich meals and promoting low-fat dairy products.

The adherents of the Mediterranean diet choose plant-based protein sources, such as beans, nuts, and seeds, which can also supply the required dietary fiber.

Antioxidants are vital for preventing or delaying cell damage, as shown.

You should choose vegetables and fruits from throughout the color spectrum to manage inflammation and give consistent energy.

In addition to numerous minerals and vitamins, vital fatty acids, dietary fiber, and beneficial phytonutrients, an anti-inflammatory diet should include a variety of minerals and vitamins.

In addition, adhering to an anti-inflammatory diet can aid in the prevention of obesity. An anti-inflammatory diet discourages the consumption of extra calories, which can result in the formation of fatty tissue and lead to obesity.

In numerous ways, an inflammatory diet and obesity may coincide. The inflammatory diet entails consuming more refined carbs, processed meats, and unhealthy foods.

Due to the low-calorie content and lack of fiber in these meals, a person will have to eat more than required to compensate for the lack of calories and sense of fullness.

Two, a person who consumes an inflammatory diet may spend more time sat and indoors, which unwittingly encourages the individual to consume more and move less.

Notably, an anti-inflammatory diet can aid in managing inflammatory disorders in already afflicted people.

Anti-inflammatory urges to eliminate refined carbohydrates and starches, for instance, can lead to type 2 diabetes, metabolic syndrome, and obesity.

Instead, the anti-inflammatory diet promotes the intake of whole grains, such as brown rice, which is high in fiber and low in glycemic load. In this way, subscribing to an anti-inflammatory diet improves a person's health over the long run.

An anti-inflammatory diet recommends consuming less saturated and trans fatty acids and more omega-3 fatty acids. Consuming unhealthy fats has been linked to an increased risk of cardiovascular disease.

One of the negative impacts of unhealthy fats is their deposition on the walls of blood vessels, which narrows them and raises blood pressure.

Increased blood pressure can cause harm to blood vessels and other organs that must adapt to a higher blood flow rate than usual. The anti-inflammatory diet recommendation encourages using heart-healthy oils like olive oil and flaxseed.

The anti-inflammatory diet can reduce blood pressure accordingly. Because it contains fewer refined carbs and harmful fats, an anti-inflammatory diet can help you lose weight.

In addition, an anti-inflammatory diet means that consuming nutrient-dense foods reduces the urge to overeat, all of which lead to unhealthy weight gain and obesity.

The consumption of complete, unprocessed meals also contributes to satiety and prevents overeating, which can lead to weight gain.

Fat accumulation in the blood arteries will eventually cause constriction and high blood pressure. Most processed foods contain salt as a preservative, and a high diet of table salt raises blood pressure.

In light of this, an anti-inflammatory diet is essential for long-term blood pressure management. an anti-inflammatory diet might decrease tiredness.

Any inflammation indicates immune system activation. When the immune system is fully engaged, histamine levels rise, causing a person to feel fatigued, weary, and irritable.

It is believed that exhaustion caused by the operations of the immune system requires slowing down and conserving energy. It is also considered that fatigue encourages rest and healing before further taxing the body.

An anti-inflammatory diet reduces or eliminates inflammation, hence eliminating or reducing the effects of the immune system that produce weariness.

A non-obesity-related benefit of an anti-inflammatory diet is weight loss. Even if you are not obese, you may be overweight or on the verge of obesity.

Other non-dietary factors, such as sedentary lifestyles, are blamed for unintentional weight gain and high consumption of refined carbs and sweets.

Refined carbohydrate foods are typically deficient in nutrients, requiring excessive consumption to meet caloric needs. In addition, refined carbohydrate foods lack fiber, resulting in a lack of satiety and excessive consumption compared to body size.

Fortunately, an anti-inflammatory diet excludes refined carbs and promotes consuming other nutrient-dense foods, meaning harmful sugars and carbohydrates are restricted.

There are additional indirect advantages to following an anti-inflammatory diet. One of these benefits is that a person will feel more at ease due to dietary choices that reduce inflammation. Inflammation manifests itself through pain, tiredness, swelling, and immobility.

According to this viewpoint, inflammation might result in absences from the job or school.

Inflammation can cause discomfort at work or school, resulting in difficulty concentrating.

By eliminating dietary inflammatory factors, a person will have a greater chance of achieving the required concentration level at work or school.

A diet low in inflammation can enhance restful sleep. Diet can contribute in numerous ways to poor sleep quality or an irregular sleep pattern.

A diet that causes inflammation will make it difficult for you to sleep regularly and be of poor quality when you do. An inflammatory diet can result in eating problems, such as waking up at night to eat, which impairs sleep quality and length.

Due to weariness, you may require frequent short naps, which will disrupt your nighttime sleep. Fortunately, an anti-inflammatory diet can eliminate dietary factors contributing to poor sleep by reducing inflammation and maintaining enough caloric and nutritional intake. Finally, an anti-inflammatory diet provides diversity and choice, allowing it to be included in other diets.

An anti-inflammatory diet is a generic term for any diet that reduces or eliminates inflammation while still providing the necessary foods and calories.

The anti-inflammatory diet encompasses a variety of diets, including vegan and Mediterranean.

By not being restricted, an anti-inflammatory diet allows individuals to make their own decisions, which is essential for the success of any dietary plan.

A diet must be flexible due to availability, affordability, cultural value, and seasonality, which influence the selection of foods.

30 DAYS DIET PLAN

DAY 1

Meal Time	Recipe	Recipe No#
Breakfast:	Turmeric Oven Scrambled Eggs	1
Lunch :	Tofu and Shrimp Capellini Soup	31
Dinner :	Vegetables Roasted with Sweet Potatoes and White Beans	61

DAY 2

Meal Time	Recipe	Recipe No#
Breakfast:	Morning Oatmeal	2
Lunch :	Salad with iceberg lettuce and mushrooms	32
Dinner :	Greens and roasted tofu	62

DAY 3

Meal Time	Recipe	Recipe No#
Breakfast:	Smoothie with blueberry	3
Lunch :	Dressed Arugula with Gorgonzola	33
Dinner :	Summer Vegetables with Italian Seasoning and Tofu	63

<table>
<tr><td colspan="3" align="center">DAY 4</td></tr>
<tr><td>Meal Time</td><td>Recipe</td><td>Recipe No#</td></tr>
<tr><td>Breakfast:</td><td>Breakfast Oatmeal</td><td>4</td></tr>
<tr><td>Lunch :</td><td>Grape Tomato and Kale Fusilli</td><td>34</td></tr>
<tr><td>Dinner :</td><td>Broccoli, Cauliflower, and Tofu with Red Onion Spice</td><td>64</td></tr>
</table>

<table>
<tr><td colspan="3" align="center">DAY 5</td></tr>
<tr><td>Meal Time</td><td>Recipe</td><td>Recipe No#</td></tr>
<tr><td>Breakfast:</td><td>Frittata with Quinoa and Asparagus Mushrooms</td><td>5</td></tr>
<tr><td>Lunch :</td><td>Pot with Rice and Chicken</td><td>35</td></tr>
<tr><td>Dinner :</td><td>Baked Tempeh and Root Vegetables</td><td>65</td></tr>
</table>

DAY 6		
Meal Time	**Recipe**	**Recipe No#**
Breakfast:	Smoothie made with cherries and spinach	6
Lunch :	Salad of Cabbage and Orange with Citrusy Vinaigrette	36
Dinner :	Chicken with Garlic and Vegetables	66

DAY 7		
Meal Time	**Recipe**	**Recipe No#**
Breakfast:	Golden Milk Chia Pudding	7
Lunch :	Rice with Lemon Butter Shrimp	37
Dinner :	Chicken with Turmeric-Spiced Sweet Potatoes, Apple, and Onion	67

DAY 8		
Meal Time	**Recipe**	**Recipe No#**
Breakfast:	No-Bake Turmeric Protein Donuts	8
Lunch :	Salad de Valencia	38
Dinner :	Carrots with honey-roasted chicken thighs	68

DAY 9		
Meal Time	**Recipe**	**Recipe No#**
Breakfast:	Choco-Nana Pancakes	9
Lunch :	Stir-Fry Tenderloin with Red and Green Grapes	39
Dinner :	Baked Sesame-Tamari Chicken with Green Beans	69

<table>
<tr><th colspan="3" align="center">DAY 10</th></tr>
<tr><th align="center">Meal Time</th><th align="center">Recipe</th><th align="center">Recipe No#</th></tr>
<tr><td>Breakfast:</td><td align="center">Bars made with Sweet Potato and Cranberries for breakfast</td><td align="center">10</td></tr>
<tr><td>Lunch :</td><td align="center">Eggs in Aioli</td><td align="center">40</td></tr>
<tr><td>Dinner :</td><td align="center">Turkey Breast on a Sheet Pan with Golden Vegetables</td><td align="center">70</td></tr>
</table>

<table>
<tr><th colspan="3" align="center">DAY 11</th></tr>
<tr><th align="center">Meal Time</th><th align="center">Recipe</th><th align="center">Recipe No#</th></tr>
<tr><td>Breakfast:</td><td align="center">Eggs scrambled with smoked salmon</td><td align="center">11</td></tr>
<tr><td>Lunch :</td><td align="center">Spaghetti Squash with Aioli</td><td align="center">41</td></tr>
<tr><td>Dinner :</td><td align="center">Steak on a Sheet Pan with Brussels Sprouts and Red Wine</td><td align="center">71</td></tr>
</table>

<table>
<tr><th colspan="3" align="center">DAY 12</th></tr>
<tr><th align="center">Meal Time</th><th align="center">Recipe</th><th align="center">Recipe No#</th></tr>
<tr><td>Breakfast:</td><td>Savory Pancakes for Breakfast</td><td>12</td></tr>
<tr><td>Lunch :</td><td>Stew with Ginger Chicken</td><td>42</td></tr>
<tr><td>Dinner :</td><td>Green Beans and Miso Salmon</td><td>72</td></tr>
</table>

DAY 13

Meal Time	Recipe	Recipe No#
Breakfast:	Smoothie made with raspberry and grapefruit	13
Lunch :	Taro with Coconut Sauce	43
Dinner :	Tilapia and Asparagus with Acorn Squash	73

DAY 14

Meal Time	Recipe	Recipe No#
Breakfast:	Breakfast Burgers on Buns Made with Avocado	14
Lunch :	Salmon Steak with Herbs de Provence	44
Dinner :	Baked Shrimp-Lime Zucchini and Corn	74

DAY 15

Meal Time	Recipe	Recipe No#
Breakfast:	Spinach Mushroom Omelet	15
Lunch :	Salad with Smoked Salmon	45
Dinner :	Broccoli and Almonds	75

DAY 16		
Meal Time	**Recipe**	**Recipe No#**
Breakfast:	Kale Turmeric Scramble	16
Lunch :	Couscous Pilaf with Turkey	46
Dinner :	Tilapia with Rosemary Pecan Topping	76

DAY 17		
Meal Time	**Recipe**	**Recipe No#**
Breakfast:	Toast with poached salmon eggs	17
Lunch :	Broccoli with anchovies and almonds	47
Dinner :	Trout Steamed with Red Bean and Chili Salsa	77

<table>
<tr><td colspan="3" align="center">DAY 18</td></tr>
<tr><td align="center">Meal Time</td><td align="center">Recipe</td><td align="center">Recipe No#</td></tr>
<tr><td>Breakfast:</td><td>Egg muffins, including feta cheese and quinoa</td><td>18</td></tr>
<tr><td>Lunch :</td><td>Stuffed Peppers with Amaranth and Quinoa</td><td>48</td></tr>
<tr><td>Dinner :</td><td>Ratatouille</td><td>78</td></tr>
</table>

DAY 19		
Meal Time	**Recipe**	**Recipe No#**
Breakfast:	Honey Almond Ricotta Peaches	19
Lunch :	Garlic and Parsley Dressed Grilled Ocean Trout	49
Dinner :	Stuffed Italian Peppers	79

DAY 20		
Meal Time	**Recipe**	**Recipe No#**
Breakfast:	Bowl of quinoa for breakfast	20
Lunch :	Sandwich with Smashed Chickpea Avocado Salad and Cranberries	50
Dinner :	Salmon with Lemon Herbs and Zucchini	80

DAY 21		
Meal Time	**Recipe**	**Recipe No#**
Breakfast:	Toast with Cream Cheese and Salmon	21
Lunch :	Delicious tuna Salad	51
Dinner :	Burgers with Sweet Potato and Black Beans	81

<table>
<tr><td colspan="3" align="center">DAY 22</td></tr>
<tr><td>Meal Time</td><td align="center">Recipe</td><td>Recipe No#</td></tr>
<tr><td>Breakfast:</td><td align="center">Carrot Cake Overnight Oats</td><td align="center">22</td></tr>
<tr><td>Lunch :</td><td align="center">Chili with Turkey</td><td align="center">52</td></tr>
<tr><td>Dinner :</td><td align="center">Stuffed Peppers with Turkey and Quinoa</td><td align="center">82</td></tr>
</table>

<table>
<tr><td colspan="3" align="center">DAY 23</td></tr>
<tr><td>Meal Time</td><td align="center">Recipe</td><td>Recipe No#</td></tr>
<tr><td>Breakfast:</td><td align="center">Mediterranean Frittata</td><td align="center">23</td></tr>
<tr><td>Lunch :</td><td align="center">Wrapped Kale Caesar Salad with Grilled Chicken</td><td align="center">53</td></tr>
<tr><td>Dinner :</td><td align="center">Zoodles with Avocado Pesto and Salmon</td><td align="center">83</td></tr>
</table>

DAY 24		
Meal Time	**Recipe**	**Recipe No#**
Breakfast:	Breakfast Chia Pudding	25
Lunch :	Egg Salad for Healthy Eating	55
Dinner :	Stir-Fry with Chicken and Snap Peas	85

DAY 26		
Meal Time	**Recipe**	**Recipe No#**
Breakfast:	Tomato Omelet	26
Lunch :	Fruit Salad in the Winter	56
Dinner :	Chicken Balsamic	86

DAY 25		
Meal Time	**Recipe**	**Recipe No#**
Breakfast:	Maple Oatmeal	24
Lunch :	Tilapia Baked with Pecan Rosemary Topping	54
Dinner :	Cakes with Salmon	84

DAY 27		
Meal Time	**Recipe**	**Recipe No#**
Breakfast:	Crockpot French Toast Casserole	27
Lunch :	Salad with Salmon Made Simple	57
Dinner :	Fried Pineapple Rice	87

<table>
<tr><td colspan="3" align="center">DAY 28</td></tr>
<tr><td>Meal Time</td><td>Recipe</td><td>Recipe No#</td></tr>
<tr><td>Breakfast:</td><td>False Banana Foster</td><td>28</td></tr>
<tr><td>Lunch :</td><td>Salad with Pasta</td><td>58</td></tr>
<tr><td>Dinner :</td><td>Roasted Chicken with Turmeric and Fennel</td><td>88</td></tr>
</table>

<table>
<tr><td colspan="3" align="center">DAY 29</td></tr>
<tr><td>Meal Time</td><td>Recipe</td><td>Recipe No#</td></tr>
<tr><td>Breakfast:</td><td>Bowl of Chicken and Quinoa Burritos</td><td>29</td></tr>
<tr><td>Lunch :</td><td>Salad with Spinach and Beans</td><td>59</td></tr>
<tr><td>Dinner :</td><td>Salmon Roasted with Potatoes and Romaine</td><td>89</td></tr>
</table>

<table>
<tr><td colspan="3" align="center">DAY 30</td></tr>
<tr><td>Meal Time</td><td>Recipe</td><td>Recipe No#</td></tr>
<tr><td>Breakfast:</td><td>Blueberry Banana Oatmeal</td><td>30</td></tr>
<tr><td>Lunch :</td><td>Salad with Kale</td><td>60</td></tr>
<tr><td>Dinner :</td><td>Soup with Chicken and Gluten-Free Noodles</td><td>90</td></tr>
</table>

CHAPTER 3

BREAKFAST RECIPE

1 Recipe for Turmeric Oven Scrambled Eggs:

Time required for preparation: 10 minutes

Cooking Time: 15 minutes

Servings: 6

Ingredients:

- ✓ 8 to 10 big pasture-raised eggs
- ✓ 1/2 cup unsweetened coconut or almond milk
- ✓ 0.5 grams of turmeric powder
- ✓ 1 milligram of chopped cilantro
- ✓ 1/4 milligram black pepper
- ✓ A grain of salt

Directions:

Preheat the oven to 3500 degrees Fahrenheit. Grease a casserole dish or an ovenproof dish. Whisk the egg, milk, turmeric powder, black pepper, and salt together in a bowl. Pour the egg mixture into the prepared baking dish and bake for 15 minutes. Remove from heat, then garnish with chopped cilantro.

Nutrition:

- ✓ Calories 203
- ✓ Total Fat 16g
- ✓ Total Carbs 5g
- ✓ Protein 10g
- ✓ Sugar: 4g
- ✓ Fiber: 1g
- ✓ Sodium: 303 mg

2 Morning Oatmeal:

Time required for preparation: 5 minutes

Cooking Time: 8 minutes

Servings: 1

Ingredients:

- ✓ 2/3 cup coconut milk
- ✓ 1 egg white from pastured chickens 12 cup gluten
- ✓ -free oats with a rapid cooking time
- ✓ 0.5 grams of turmeric powder
- ✓ 0.5 grams cinnamon
- ✓ 1/4 milligram ginger

Direction:

Prepare the nondairy milk by placing it in a pot and heating it over a medium temperature. Incorporate the egg white and continue whisking until a smooth consistency is achieved. Add the other ingredients and simmer for an additional three minutes.

Nutrition:

- ✓ Calories 395
- ✓ Total Fat 34g
- ✓ Total Carbs 19g
- ✓ Protein 10g
- ✓ Sugar: 2g
- ✓ Fiber: 3g
- ✓ Sodium: 76mg

3 Smoothies with blueberry

Time required for preparation: 5 minutes

Cooking Time: 0 minutes

Servings: 1

Ingredients

- ✓ 1 cup almond milk ingredients
- ✓ 1 frozen banana

- ✓ 1 volume of frozen blueberries
- ✓ 2 bunches of spinach
- ✓ 1 gram of almond butter
- ✓ 1/4 milligram cinnamon
- ✓ 1/4 teaspoon chili pepper
- ✓ 1 teaspoon maca powder

Instructions:

 Pulse all the ingredients in a blender until thoroughly incorporated. Serve without delay.

Nutrition:

- ✓ Calories 431
- ✓ Protein 10g
- ✓ Total Fat 21g
- ✓ Total Carbs 56g
- ✓ Net Carbs 48g
- ✓ Sugar: 38g
- ✓ Fiber: 8g
- ✓ Sodium: 201mg

4 Breakfast Oatmeal:

Time Required for Preparation: 15 minutes

Cooking Time: 0 minutes

Servings: 1

Ingredients:

- ✓ 6 teaspoons natural cottage cheese
- ✓ Three tablespoons of flaxseed
- ✓ three teaspoons of flax oil
- ✓ two tablespoons of organic raw almond butter.
- ✓ 1 teaspoon natural coconut flesh
- ✓ 1 teaspoon natural honey
- ✓ 1/4 cup water

Direction:

Combine all of the ingredients in a bowl. Mix until well mixed. Place in a bowl and refrigerate before serving.

Nutrition:

- ✓ Calories 632
- ✓ 49g total fat
- ✓ 32g total carbohydrates
- ✓ 26g net carbohydrates
- ✓ Sugar: 22g
- ✓ Fiber: 6g

✓ Sodium: 265mg

5 Frittata with Quinoa and Asparagus Mushrooms:

Time required for preparation: 5 minutes

Cooking Time: 30 minutes

Servings: 3

Ingredients:

✓ 2 tablespoons olive oil

✓ 1 quart of sliced mushrooms

✓ 1 cup of asparagus sliced into 1-inch lengths

✓ 12 cups diced tomato

✓ 6 big eggs, pasture-raised

✓ 2 big pasture-raised egg whites 14 cups nondairy milk

✓ 1 cup quinoa cooked according to the instructions on the box

✓ 3 teaspoons minced basil

✓ 1 tablespoon of chopped parsley

✓ season to taste with salt and pepper

Directions:

Preheat the oven to 3500 degrees Fahrenheit. Warm the olive oil over the medium temperature in a skillet. Stir in the mushrooms and asparagus, then season to taste with salt and pepper. For seven minutes, sauté the mushrooms and asparagus until they have browned. Cook the tomatoes for a further 3 minutes. Set aside. In the meantime, combine the eggs, egg white, and milk in a dish. Set aside. Place the quinoa in a baking dish and cover it with the veggie mixture. Incorporate the egg mixture. Bake for 20 minutes or until the eggs have solidified.

Nutrition:

- ✓ Calories 450
- ✓ 37g of total fat
- ✓ 17g of total carbs
- ✓ 14g of net carbs
- ✓ 12g of protein
- ✓ Sugar: 2g
- ✓ Fiber: 3g
- ✓ Sodium: 60mg

6 Smoothie made with cherries and spinach.

Time required for preparation: 5 minutes

Cooking Time: 0 minutes

Servings: 1

Ingredients:

- ✓ 1 cup of simple kefir
- ✓ 1 cup frozen, pitted cherries
- ✓ 12 cups baby spinach leaves
- ✓ 14 cups ripe avocado mashed
- ✓ 1 gram of almond butter
- ✓ 1-piece peeled ginger (1/2 inch)
- ✓ a tablespoon of chia seeds

Directions:

Put all of the ingredients into a blender. Pulse till creamy. Allow cooling in the refrigerator before serving.

Nutrition:

- ✓ Calories 410
- ✓ 20g total fat
- ✓ 47g total carbohydrates
- ✓ 37g net carbohydrates 17g

✓ Sugar: 33g

✓ Fiber: 10g

✓ Sodium: 169mg

7 Golden Milk Chia Pudding:

Time required for preparation: 6 hours

Cooking Time: 0 minutes

Servings: 4

Ingredients:

✓ Four pints of coconut milk

✓ 3 teaspoons of honey

✓ 1 teaspoon vanilla essence

✓ 2 teaspoons turmeric powder

✓ 1/2 teaspoon cinnamon powder

✓ 1/2 teaspoon ginger powder

✓ quarter cup coconut yogurt

✓ ½ cup chia seeds

✓ 1 cup of assorted fresh berries

✓ ¼ cup toasted coconut chips

Directions:

In a mixing dish, combine the coconut milk, honey, vanilla essence, turmeric, cinnamon, and ginger. Incorporate the coconut yogurt. Place chia seeds, berries, and coconut chips in bowls. Incorporate the milk mixture. Allow six hours of chilling in the refrigerator for setting.

Nutrition:

- ✓ Calories 337
- ✓ 11g total fat
- ✓ 51g total carbohydrates
- ✓ 10g protein
- ✓ Sugar: 29g
- ✓ Fiber: 2g
- ✓ Sodium: 262mg

8 No-Bake Turmeric Protein Donuts:

Time for Preparation: 50 minutes

Cooking Time: 0 minutes

Servings: 8

Ingredients:

- ✓ 1.5 cups uncooked cashews
- ✓ 12 cup pitted Medjool dates
- ✓ 1 tbsp vanilla protein powder
- ✓ 1/2 cup grated coconut
- ✓ 2 tablespoons maple syrup
- ✓ ¼ teaspoon vanilla extract
- ✓ 1 teaspoon ground turmeric
- ✓ 1/4 cup of chocolate

Directions:

Except for the chocolate, combine all ingredients in a food processor. Pulse till creamy. Roll the batter into eight balls and press into a donut silicone form. To set, chill for 30 minutes. In the meantime, prepare the chocolate topping by melting chocolate in a double boiler. After the donuts have hardened, take them from the mold and sprinkle them with chocolate.

Nutrition:

- ✓ Calories 320
- ✓ 26g Total Fat
- ✓ 20g Total Carbohydrates
- ✓ 7g Protein

- ✓ Sugar: 9g
- ✓ Fiber: 2g
- ✓ Sodium:163 mg

9 Choco-Nana Pancakes:

Time required for preparation: 5 minutes

Cooking Time: 6 minutes

Servings: 2

Ingredients:
- ✓ 2 big peeled and mashed bananas
- ✓ 2 big eggs, pasture-raised
- ✓ 3 tbsp cacao powder
- ✓ 2 tablespoons of almond spread
- ✓ 1 teaspoon pure vanilla essence
- ✓ 1/8 teaspoon salt
- ✓ Coconut oil as a lubricant

Directions:

Warm a skillet over medium-low heat while greasing it with coconut oil. Place all ingredients in a food processor and pulse until completely combined. Pour around 14 cups of batter into the skillet to produce a pancake. Cook for three minutes per side.

Nutrition:

- ✓ Calories 303
- ✓ 17g Total Fat
- ✓ 36g Total Carbohydrates
- ✓ 5g Protein
- ✓ Sugar: 15g
- ✓ Fiber: 5g
- ✓ Sodium: 108mg

10 Bars made with Sweet Potato and Cranberries for breakfast:

Time required for preparation: 10 minutes

Cooking Time: 40 minutes

Servings: 8

Ingredients:

- ✓ 1 1/2 cups pureed sweet potato
- ✓ 2 tablespoons coconut oil, melted

- ✓ 2 tablespoons maple syrup
- ✓ 2 eggs, pasture-raised
- ✓ 1 cup almond meal
- ✓ 1/3 cup coconut flour
- ✓ 1 ½ teaspoon baking soda
- ✓ 1 cup fresh, pitted, and diced cranberries
- ✓ 1/4 cup water

Directions:

Preheat the oven to 3500 degrees Fahrenheit. Coconut oil is used to grease a baking sheet. Set aside. In a mixing dish, combine the sweet potato puree, water, coconut oil, maple syrup, and eggs. Sift the coconut flour, baking soda, and almond flour into a separate dish. Place the dry fastener onto the wet fastener. Mix. Place in the baking dish and top with the cranberries. Bake for 40 minutes or until a toothpick inserted into the center of the cake comes out clean. Before removing it from the pan, allow it to rest or cool.

Nutrition:

- ✓ Calories 98
- ✓ 6g total fat
- ✓ 9g total carbohydrates
- ✓ 3g protein

- ✓ Sugar: 7g
- ✓ Fiber: 0.5g
- ✓ Sodium:113 mg

11 Eggs scrambled with smoked salmon:

Time required for preparation: 10 minutes

Cooking Time: 10 minutes

Servings: 2

Ingredients:
- ✓ 4 eggs
- ✓ 2 tablespoons coconut milk
- ✓ Fresh chopped chives
- ✓ 4 slices of wild-caught smoked salmon
- ✓ to taste with chopped salt

Directions:

Whisk together the egg, coconut milk, and chives in a bowl. Apply oil to the skillet and heat over medium-low heat. Place the egg mixture, then scramble it while it cooks. When the eggs begin to settle, add the smoked salmon and continue cooking for an additional two minutes.

Nutrition:

- ✓ Calories 349
- ✓ 23g Total Fat
- ✓ 3g Total Carbohydrates
- ✓ 29g Protein
- ✓ Sugar: 2g Fiber: 2g
- ✓ Sodium: 466mg

12 Savory Pancakes for Breakfast:

Time required for preparation: 5 minutes

Cooking Time: 6 minutes

Servings: 4

Ingredients:

- ✓ ½ cup almond flour
- ✓ ½ cup tapioca flour
- ✓ 1 fluid ounce of coconut milk
- ✓ 0.5 grams of chili powder
- ✓ 1/4 teaspoon ground turmeric
- ✓ 12 red onions, minced 1 handful of cilantro leaves

- ✓ minced 12 inches of grated ginger
- ✓ 1 teaspoon salt
- ✓ 1/4 teaspoon black pepper

Directions:

In a bowl, blend all the ingredients until well-combined. Oil a pan and cook it over low to medium heat while greasing it with oil. Pour a quarter cup of batter onto the pan and spread it out to form a pancake. Fry for 3 minutes per side.

Nutrition:

- ✓ Calories 108
- ✓ 2g Total Fat
- ✓ 20g Total Carbohydrates
- ✓ 2g Protein
- ✓ Sugar: 4g
- ✓ Fiber: 0.5g
- ✓ Sodium: 37mg
- ✓ Potassium 95mg

13 Smoothies made with raspberry and grapefruit:

Time required for preparation: 5 minutes

Cooking Time: 0 minutes

Servings: 1

Ingredients:

- ✓ Freshly squeezed grapefruit juice
- ✓ 1 banana
- ✓ peeled and sliced 1 cup raspberries

Directions:

Blend the ingredients in a blender until smooth. Before serving, chill.

Nutrition:

- ✓ Calories 381
- ✓ Total Fat 0.8g
- ✓ Net Carbohydrates 96g
- ✓ Protein 4g
- ✓ Sugar: 61g
- ✓ Fiber: 11g
- ✓ Sodium: 11mg
- ✓ Potassium 848mg

14 Breakfast Burgers on Buns Made with Avocado:

Time required for preparation: 10 minutes

Cooking Time: 5 minutes

Servings: 1

Ingredients:

- ✓ 1 ripe avocado
- ✓ 1 egg, pasture-raised
- ✓ a single onion slice
- ✓ 1 tomato slice
- ✓ 1 lettuce leaf
- ✓ To garnish with sesame seeds
- ✓ salt to taste

Directions:

Halve the avocado lengthwise. It will function like bread. Set aside. Grease a pan and cook the egg sunny-side over a medium temperature for five minutes or until set.Assemble the morning burger by arranging the egg, red onion, tomato, and lettuce leaf on top of one avocado half. Add the remaining avocado bun on top.The dish should be topped with sesame seeds and salted to taste.

Nutrition:

- ✓ Calories 458
- ✓ Total Fat 39g
- ✓ Total Carbs 20g

- ✓ Protein 13g S

- ✓ sugar: 8g

- ✓ Fiber: 14g

15 Spinach Mushroom Omelet:

Time to Prepare: 3 minutes

Cooking Time: 15 minutes

Servings: 2

Ingredients:
- ✓ Olive oil

- ✓ one tablespoon of Fresh spinach chopped

- ✓ 1 and 1/2 cups Green onion diced

- ✓ 1 Egg

- ✓ three Feta cheese

- ✓ one-ounce button mushrooms

- ✓ five sliced, chopped red onion

- ✓ a quarter cup of red wine vinegar.

Directions:

Three minutes later, sauté the mushrooms, onions, and spinach in one tablespoon of olive oil and leave aside. Beat the eggs thoroughly and fry them for three to four minutes in the remaining tablespoon of olive oil until the edges begin to brown. On one side of the omelet, sprinkle the remaining ingredients, then fold the other half over the sautéed contents. Prepare for one minute per side.

Nutrition:
- ✓ Calories 337
- ✓ fat 25 grams
- ✓ protein 22 grams
- ✓ carbohydrates 5.4 grams
- ✓ sugar 1.3 grams
- ✓ fiber 1-gram

16 Kale Turmeric Scramble:

Time required for preparation: 5 minutes

Cooking Time: 10 minutes

Servings: 1

Ingredients:
- ✓ olive oil
- ✓ two tablespoons of shredded kale
- ✓ one-half cup of sprouts

- ✓ one tablespoon of minced garlic
- ✓ one-quarter teaspoon of ground turmeric
- ✓ and one tablespoon of ground black pepper
- ✓ Eggs two

Directions:

Incorporate turmeric, black pepper, and garlic into the beaten eggs. Five minutes after sautéing the kale in olive oil over medium heat, pour this egg batter into the pan with the kale. Continue to cook, frequently stirring, until the eggs are cooked. Serve with raw sprouts on top.

Nutrition:

- ✓ Calories 137
- ✓ fat 8.4 grams
- ✓ carbohydrates 7.9 grams
- ✓ fiber 4.8 grams
- ✓ sugar 1.8grams
- ✓ protein 13.2 grams

17 Toast with poached salmon eggs:

Time required for preparation: 10 minutes

Cooking Time: 4 minutes

Servings: 2

Ingredients:

- ✓ Toasted rye or whole-grain bread
- ✓ two slices of Lemon juice
- ✓ a quarter teaspoon of mashed avocado
- ✓ two teaspoons of Black pepper
- ✓ one-fourth teaspoon Eggs
- ✓ two poached Smoked salmon
- ✓ four ounces Scallions
- ✓ one teaspoon of thinly sliced
- ✓ one-eighth teaspoon of salt

Directions:

Add lemon juice, pepper, and salt to the avocado. Spread the avocado mixture on the toasted bread. On bread, place smoked salmon and a poached egg. Finished with sliced scallions.

Nutrition:

- ✓ 389 calories
- ✓ Fat 17.2 grams
- ✓ Protein 33.5 grams
- ✓ Carbohydrates 31.5 grams
- ✓ sugar1.3 grams
- ✓ fiber 9.3 grams

18 Egg muffins, including feta cheese and quinoa:

Time Required for Preparation: 15 minutes

Cooking Time: 30 minutes

Servings: 12

Ingredients:

- ✓ Eggs
- ✓ eight chopped tomatoes
- ✓ one cup salt
- ✓ one-fourth teaspoon of feta cheese
- ✓ one cup of cooked quinoa
- ✓ one cup of olive oil
- ✓ two teaspoons of chopped fresh oregano
- ✓ one tablespoon of chopped fresh black olives
- ✓ and one-fourth cup of chopped onion
- ✓ chopped baby spinach, two cups

Directions:

Preheat oven to 350 degrees Fahrenheit. Spray a muffin tin with twelve cups of oil. Cook spinach, oregano, olives, onion, and tomatoes in olive oil over medium heat for five minutes. Beat eggs. Add the cooked vegetable mixture, cheese, and salt to the eggs.

Place the mixture in muffin cups. Bake for 30 minutes. These will keep fresh for two days in the refrigerator. To consume, wrap in a paper towel and microwave for thirty seconds.

Nutrition:
- ✓ Calorie 113
- ✓ carbohydrates 5 grams
- ✓ protein 6 grams
- ✓ fat 7 grams
- ✓ sugar 1-gram

19 Honey Almond Ricotta Peaches:

Time Required for Preparation: 15 minutes

Cooking Time: 0 minutes

Servings: 6

Ingredients:
- ✓ Ricotta
- ✓ skim milk
- ✓ one cup of honey
- ✓ one teaspoon of sliced almonds
- ✓ half a cup of almond essence
- ✓ a quarter teaspoon

To Provide

- ✓ One cup of sliced peaches
- ✓ Whole grain bagel or toast

Directions:

Almond extract, honey, ricotta, and almonds should be combined. On toasted bread, spread one tablespoon of this mixture and top with peaches.

Nutrition:

- ✓ Calories 230
- ✓ protein 9 grams
- ✓ fat 8 grams
- ✓ carbohydrates grams 37
- ✓ fiber 3 grams
- ✓ sugar 34 grams

20 Bowl of quinoa for breakfast:

Time to Prepare: 30 minutes

Cooking Time: 0 minutes

Servings: 6

Ingredients:

- ✓ Cooked quinoa two cups

- ✓ Eggs
- ✓ twelve Plain Greek yogurt
- ✓ a quarter cup of Sodium
- ✓ a half-teaspoon of Feta cheese
- ✓ a cup of cherry tomatoes
- ✓ and a pint of halved cherry tomatoes.
- ✓ Black pepper 1 teaspoon
- ✓ Minced garlic 1 teaspoon
- ✓ chopped baby spinach 1 cup
- ✓ Olive oil 1 teaspoon

Directions:

Eggs, salt, pepper, garlic powder, onion powder, and yogurt are combined. Cook the spinach and tomatoes for five minutes over medium heat in the olive oil. Pour in the egg mixture and whisk until the eggs have reached the desired consistency. Warm the quinoa and feta by mixing them. It can be refrigerated for two to three days.

Nutrition:

- ✓ Calories 340
- ✓ fat 7.3 grams
- ✓ carbohydrates 59.4 grams
- ✓ fiber 6.2 grams
- ✓ sugar 21.4 grams
- ✓ protein 10.5 grams

21 Toast with Cream Cheese and Salmon:

Time required for preparation: 10 minutes

Cooking Time: 2 minutes

Servings: 2

Ingredients:

- ✓ two pieces of whole grain or rye bread toast
- ✓ finely sliced red onion, two teaspoons
- ✓ Low-fat cream cheese, two teaspoons
- ✓ Basil flakes, 1/2 teaspoon Arugula
- ✓ spinach, finely cut, 1/2 cup
- ✓ Two ounces of smoked salmon

Directions:

Warm the whole wheat bread. Cream cheese and basil are combined and smeared over bread. Add salmon, arugula, and onion.

Nutrition:

- ✓ Calories 291
- ✓ fat 15.2 grams
- ✓ carbs 17.8 grams
- ✓ sugar 3 grams

22 Carrot Cake Overnight Oats:

Preparation Time: 24 hours

Cooking Time: 1 minute

Servings: 2

Ingredients:

- ✓ One cup of Chia seed
- ✓ one tablespoon of ground cinnamon
- ✓ one teaspoon of raisins
- ✓ one-half cup of low-fat cream cheese
- ✓ two tablespoons of room-temperature cream cheese.
- ✓ Carrot, a substantial peel, and shred
- ✓ two teaspoons Vanilla
- ✓ two tablespoons honey

Directions:

Combine all of the ingredients and refrigerate them overnight in a secure container. Consume cold foods in the morning. If you wish to reheat this dish, microwave it for one minute and toss it before serving.

Nutrition:

- ✓ Calories 340

- ✓ sugar 32 grams

- ✓ protein 8 grams

- ✓ fat 4 grams

- ✓ fiber 9 grams

- ✓ carbohydrates 70 grams

23 Mediterranean Frittata:

Time required for preparation: 5 minutes

Cooking Time: 20 minutes

Servings: 6

Ingredients:

- ✓ Eggs

- ✓ six crumbled Feta cheese

- ✓ a quarter cup of black pepper

- ✓ and a quarter teaspoon of oil

- ✓ spritz

- ✓ olive oil.

- ✓ Oregano

- ✓ one teaspoon Milk

- ✓ almond or coconut one-fourth cup

✓ Sea salt one teaspoon

✓ Chopped black olives,one-fourth cup

✓ Chopped green olives, one-fourth cup

✓ Diced tomatoes, one-fourth cup

Directions:

Preheat oven to 400 degrees Fahrenheit. Prepare one eight-by-eight-inch baking dish with cooking oil. Combine the milk and eggs, then add the other ingredients. This mixture should be poured into the baking dish and baked for twenty minutes.

Nutrition:

✓ Calories 107

✓ sugars 2 grams

✓ fat 7 grams

✓ carb 3 grams

protein 7 grams

24 Maple Oatmeal:

Time required for preparation: 5 minutes

Cooking Time: 20 minutes

Servings: 4

Ingredients:

- ✓ Flavoring of maple syrup
- ✓ one teaspoon cinnamon
- ✓ one teaspoon of sunflower seeds
- ✓ three tablespoons pecans
- ✓ one-half cup chopped unsweetened coconut flakes
- ✓ one-fourth cup walnuts
- ✓ one-half cup chopped almond
- ✓ coconut milk one-half cup
- ✓ Chia seeds four teaspoons.

Directions:

Grind the sunflower seeds, walnuts, and pecans into crumbs in a food processor. Alternatively, you may place the nuts in a durable plastic bag, cover the bag in a towel, set it on a firm surface, and pound the towel with a hammer until the nuts are broken up. Pour the crushed nuts and the remaining ingredients into a big saucepan after combining them. This mixture should simmer for thirty minutes over low heat. Stir often, so the bottom does not stick. If desired, serve with fresh fruit or a dusting of cinnamon.

Nutrition:

- ✓ Calories 374
- ✓ carbohydrates 3.2 grams
- ✓ protein 9.25 grams

✓ fat 34.59 grams

25 Tomato Omelet:

Time Required for Preparation: 20 minutes

Cooking Time: 8 minutes

Servings: 1

Ingredients:

✓ two eggs

✓ two fresh basil leaves

✓ half a cup of cherry tomatoes

✓ half a cup of black pepper

✓ a quarter cup of any shredded cheese

✓ Sodium 0.5 teaspoon

✓ Olive oil two teaspoons

Directions:

The tomatoes are quartered. Fry it for three minutes in olive oil. Place the tomatoes on one side. Add salt and pepper to the eggs in a small bowl, then thoroughly combine. Pour the beaten egg mixture into the pan and use a spatula to work around the omelet's borders carefully; then, let the eggs cook for three minutes without stirring. Add basil, tomatoes, and cheese while the center third of the egg mixture is still liquid. Half of the omelet is folded over the other half. Cook for two minutes longer, then serve.

Nutrition:

- ✓ Calories 342
- ✓ carbohydrates 8 grams
- ✓ protein 20 grams
- ✓ fat 25.3 grams

26 Breakfast Chia Pudding:

Time to Prepare: 3 minutes

Cooking Time: 0 minutes

Servings: 2

Ingredients:

- ✓ Chia seeds
- ✓ four tablespoons of almond butter
- ✓ one tablespoon of coconut milk
- ✓ three-quarters of a cup of cinnamon
- ✓ one teaspoon of vanilla
- ✓ one teaspoon of cold coffee
- ✓ three-quarters of a cu

Direction:

Combine all the condiments and pour them into a jar that can be stored in the refrigerator. Cover well and chill overnight.

Nutrition:

- ✓ Calories 282
- ✓ scarabs 5 grams
- ✓ protein 5.9 grams
- ✓ fat 24 grams

27 Crockpot French Toast Casserole:

Time Required for Preparation: 15 minutes

Time Required: 4 hours

Servings: 9

Ingredients:

- ✓ 2 eggs
- ✓ 2 beaten egg whites
- ✓ 1 ½ almond milk or 1% milk
- ✓ 2 tablespoons of raw honey
- ✓ 0.5 grams cinnamon
- ✓ 1 tsp vanilla extract
- ✓ 9 pieces bread

- ✓ For filling:
- ✓ 3cups apples (diced)
- ✓ 2 tablespoons of raw honey
- ✓ 1 tbsp lemon juice
- ✓ 0.5 grams cinnamon
- ✓ 0.3 ounce of pecans

Directions:

Mix the first six ingredients in a bowl. Spray the slow cooker with a cooking spray that prevents sticking. In a small dish, combine all the filling ingredients and leave aside. Coat the apple chunks properly with the filling. Cut bread pieces in half (triangle), then layer the bottom with three apple slices and filling. The bread pieces and contents are layered in the same manner. Apply the egg mixture to the bread and filling layers. Adjust the temperature to high for 2 12 hours or low for 4 hours.

Nutrition:

- ✓ Calories: 227
- ✓ Total Fat: 7g
- ✓ Carbohydrates: 34g
- ✓ Protein: 9g
- ✓ Sugar: 19g
- ✓ Fiber 4g
- ✓ Sodium: 187 mg

28 False Banana Foster:

Time Required for Preparation: 15 minutes

Time Required: 2 hours

Servings: 3

Ingredients:

- ✓ 1 tbsp melted coconut oil (unrefined)
- ✓ 3 mL of honey
- ✓ grams cinnamon
- ✓ Half of a medium-sized lemon's juice
- ✓ 5 bananas (medium-sized)
- ✓ For Seasoning:
- ✓ hacked nuts
- ✓ Greek Yogurt

Directions:

Mix the first four ingredients in a slow cooker. Halve the bananas and add them to the slow cooker's mixture. Set the cooker on low heat for between 1, 12, and 2 hours. Serve alongside chopped nuts or Greek yogurt.

Nutrition:

- ✓ Calories: 220

- ✓ Total Fat: 4g
- ✓ Carbohydrates: 56 g
- ✓ Protein: 4g
- ✓ Sugar: 36g
- ✓ Fiber 4g
- ✓ Sodium: 4 mg
- ✓ 0mg Cholesterol

29 Bowl of Chicken and Quinoa Burritos:

Time required for preparation: 10 minutes

Time Required: 5 hours

Servings: 6

Ingredients:
- ✓ 1 pound of chicken thighs (skinless, boneless)
- ✓ 1 cup chicken stock
- ✓ One may consume chopped tomatoes (14.5oz)
- ✓ 1 onion (chopped)
- ✓ 3 bulbs of garlic (chopped)
- ✓ 2 tsp chili powder
- ✓ 0.5 g coriander
- ✓ 0.5 grams of garlic powder

✓ 1 bell pepper (finely chopped)

✓ 15oz pinto beans (drained)

✓ 1 ½ cup cheddar cheese (grated)

Directions:

Mix chicken, tomatoes, broth, onion, garlic, chili powder, garlic powder, coriander, and salt. Place the stove on low heat. Using a fork and knife, shred the chicken into small pieces. Add quinoa and pinto beans to the slow cooker along with the shredded chicken. Set the heat to low for two hours. Continue to boil and stir gently until the cheese melts after adding it on top. Serve.

Nutrition:

✓ Calories: 144mg

✓ Total Fat: 39g

✓ Carbohydrates: 68 g

✓ Protein: 59g

✓ Sugar: 8g

✓ Fiber 17g

✓ Sodium: 756 mg

✓ 144 milligrams of cholesterol

30 Blueberry Banana Oatmeal

Time to Prepare: 10 minutes

Time Required: 2 hours

Servings: 6

Ingredients:
- ✓ 2 cups of rolled food
- ✓ 1/4 cup almonds (toasted)
- ✓ 1 ounce of walnuts
- ✓ 1/4 cup pecans
- ✓ 2 tablespoons ground flaxseed
- ✓ 1 tsp of ginger powder
- ✓ 1 teaspoon cinnamon
- ✓ 1/4 tsp sea salt
- ✓ 2 tbsp coconut sugar
- ✓ ½ tsp baking powder
- ✓ 2 gallons of milk
- ✓ 2 bananas
- ✓ 1 ounce of ripe blueberries
- ✓ 1 tbsp maple syrup
- ✓ 1 tsp vanilla extract
- ✓ 1 tbsp melted butter
- ✓ Yogurt for serving

Directions:

Mix coconut sugar, nuts, flax seeds, baking powder, spices, and coconut sugar in a large bowl. Whisk together eggs, milk, maple syrup, and vanilla in a separate dish. Halve the bananas and top them with blueberries in the slow cooker. On top of the oats mixture, pour the milk mixture. Drizzle with butter that has been melted. Cook the slow cooker for four hours on low heat or high heat. Cook until the liquid has been absorbed and the oats have turned golden brown. Serve warm, with plain Greek yogurt on top.

Nutrition:

- ✓ Calories: 346 mg
- ✓ Total Fat: 15g
- ✓ Carbohydrates: 45g
- ✓ Protein: 11g
- ✓ Sugar: 17g
- ✓ Fiber 7g
- ✓ Sodium: 145 mg
- ✓ cholesterol: 39 milligrams

31 Tofu and Shrimp Capellini Soup

Time to prepare: 20 minutes

Time to cook: 20 minutes

8 servings

Ingredients:

- ✓ 4 cups sliced bok choy
- ✓ 1/4 pound peeled and deveined shrimp
- ✓ 1 firm tofu block, sliced into squares
- ✓ 1 can of drained sliced water chestnuts
- ✓ 1 bunch of sliced scallions
- ✓ 2 cups chicken broth (low sodium)
- ✓ 2 teaspoons of reduced-sodium soy sauce
- ✓ capellini 2 cups
- ✓ 2 tablespoons sesame oil
- ✓ white pepper, freshly ground
- ✓ 1 tablespoon rice wine vinegar

Directions:

In a saucepan over medium-high heat, pour in the broth. Bring the water to a boil. Combine the shrimp, bok choy, oil, and sauce in a mixing bowl. Allow coming to a boil before lowering the heat. Cook for 5 minutes. Combine the water chestnuts, pepper, vinegar, tofu, capellini, and scallions in a mixing bowl. Cook for 5 minutes or until the capellini is just tender. Serve immediately.

Nutrition:

- ✓ 205 calories
- ✓ Carbohydrates: 20g
- ✓ Fat: 9g
- ✓ 9g protein

32 Salad with iceberg lettuce and mushrooms

Time to Prepare: 10 minutes

Time to cook: 20 minutes

4 servings

Ingredients:

- ✓ 1 large iceberg lettuce head, sliced into 6 equal wedges, core retained, rinsed and spun-dried
- ✓ To make the dressing
- ✓ 1 can, 15 oz. button mushroom stems and pieces, rinsed and drained thoroughly

- ✓ 1 cup plain Greek yogurt
- ✓ 1 14-cup cottage cheese
- ✓ 2 Tbsp. freshly squeezed lemon juice
- ✓ 12 cup vinegar (white)
- ✓ ½ tsp. Pepper, black
- ✓ ¼ tsp. stevia leaf

Directions:

Besides the button mushrooms, whisk together all the dressing ingredients in a mixing bowl. Mix until smooth. Add more vinegar if the dressing is too thick. Mix in the mushrooms. Divide the mixture into 6 equal parts. On a plate, place 1 lettuce wedge. 1 portion of the dressing on top

Nutrition:

- ✓ 15 calories
- ✓ 3g carbs
- ✓ Fat: 0g
- ✓ 1g protein

33 Dressed Arugula with Gorgonzola

Time to Prepare: 10 minutes

Time to cook: 0 minutes

4 servings

Ingredients:

- ✓ 1 bunch of arugula, washed
- ✓ 1 pear, thinly sliced
- ✓ 1 tablespoon freshly squeezed lemon juice
- ✓ 1 crushed garlic clove
- ✓ 1/3 cup crumbled Gorgonzola cheese
- ✓ 1/4 cup reduced-sodium vegetable stock
- ✓ pepper, freshly ground
- ✓ 4 tbsp. olive oil
- ✓ 1 tbsp apple cider vinegar

Directions:

In a mixing bowl, combine the pear slices and lemon juice. To coat, toss everything together. Arrange the pear slices and arugula on a serving platter. Combine the vinegar, oil, cheese, broth, pepper, and garlic in a mixing bowl. Remove the garlic after 5 minutes. Serve with the dressing.

Nutrition:

- ✓ 145 calories

✓ Carbohydrates: 23g

✓ Fat: 4g

✓ 6g protein

34 Grape Tomato and Kale Fusilli

Time to Prepare: 15 minutes

Time to cook: 15 minutes

4 servings

Ingredients:

✓ 14 cup wholegrain fusilli, cooked as directed on the package
✓ 1 kale handful, sliced into bite-sized pieces
✓ 12 cup quartered grape tomatoes
✓ 2 Tbsp. liquid for cooking
✓ ½ Tbsp. extra virgin olive oil
✓ 14 cups thinly sliced leeks
✓ 1 minced garlic clove
✓ 1 tsp sea salt
✓ To taste, a pinch of black pepper
✓ 1 tsp. chopped roasted almonds

✓ grated pecorino cheese for sprinkling

Directions:

Heat the oil in a saucepan over high heat. Mix in the leeks and garlic. Reduce the heat to low and cook until the leeks are soft, about 2 minutes. Mix in the kale and tomatoes. 4 minutes later, the kale should be wilted. Except for the cheese, combine the remaining ingredients. To combine, toss everything together thoroughly. Place the pasta dish on a plate and top it with pecorino cheese. Serve.

Nutrition:

✓ 510 calories

✓ Carbohydrates: 42g

✓ Fat: 32g

✓ 16g protein

35 Pot with Rice and Chicken

Time to Prepare: 5 minutes

Time to cook: 25 minutes

4 servings

Ingredients:

- ✓ 1 lb. boneless, skinless free-range chicken breast
- ✓ 14 cups brown rice
- ✓ ¾ lb. sliced mushrooms of choice
- ✓ 1 chopped leek
- ✓ 14 cups chopped almonds
- ✓ 1 quart of water
- ✓ 1 Tbsp. extra virgin olive oil
- ✓ 1 pound green beans
- ✓ 12 cups of apple cider vinegar
- ✓ 2 Tbsp. universal flour
- ✓ 1 cup of low-fat milk
- ✓ 14 cups freshly grated Parmesan cheese
- ✓ 14 cups soured cream
- ✓ a pinch of sea salt, more if desired
- ✓ to taste, ground black pepper

Directions:

Fill a pot halfway with brown rice. Pour in the water. Bring to a boil, covered. Reduce the heat to low and cook for 30 minutes or until the rice is tender. Meanwhile, season the chicken breast in a skillet with salt and pour just enough water to cover it. Bring the mixture to a boil, then reduce to low heat and allow it to simmer for 10 minutes. Chicken should be shredded. Place aside. Heat the olive oil. Cook leeks until they are tender. Mix in the mushrooms. Add the apple cider vinegar to the mixture. Cook until the vinegar has evaporated from the mixture. In the skillet, combine the flour and milk. Sprinkle with Parmesan cheese and sour cream Season with black pepper to taste. Preheat the oven to 350 degrees Fahrenheit. Grease a casserole dish lightly with oil. Spread the cooked rice in the casserole dish, followed by the shredded chicken and green beans. Sauce with mushrooms and leeks. Sprinkle with almonds. Cook for 20 minutes or until golden brown. Allow cooling before serving.

Nutrition:
- ✓ 401 calories
- ✓ Carbohydrates: 54g
- ✓ Fat: 12g
- ✓ 20g protein

36 Salad of Cabbage and Orange with Citrusy Vinaigrette

Time to Prepare: 10 minutes

Time to cook: 0 minutes

8 servings

Ingredients:

- ✓ 1 teaspoon grated orange zest

- ✓ 2 tbsp reduced-sodium vegetable stock
- ✓ 1 teaspoon of each apple cider vinegar
- ✓ 4 cups shredded red cabbage
- ✓ 1 tsp. lemon juice
- ✓ 1 fennel bulb, thinly sliced
- ✓ a tsp of balsamic vinegar
- ✓ 1 tablespoon of raspberry vinegar
- ✓ 2 tbsp freshly squeezed orange juice
- ✓ 2 oranges, peeled and sliced
- ✓ 1 teaspoon of honey
- ✓ a quarter teaspoon of salt
- ✓ pepper, freshly ground
- ✓ 4 tablespoons olive oil

Directions:

In a mixing bowl, combine the lemon juice, orange zest, cider vinegar, salt and pepper, broth, oil, honey, orange juice, balsamic vinegar, and raspberry. Oranges, fennel, and cabbage should be extracted. To coat, toss everything together.

Nutrition:

- ✓ 70 calories
- ✓ 14g carbs
- ✓ Fat: 0g
- ✓ 1g protein

37 Rice with Lemon Butter Shrimp

Time to Prepare: 15 minutes

Time to cook: 10 minutes

3 servings

Ingredients:

- ✓ 14 cups wild rice, cooked
- ✓ ½ tsp. divided butter
- ✓ ¼ tsp. extra virgin olive oil
- ✓ 1 cup shelled, deveined, and drained raw shrimp
- ✓ 14 cups frozen peas, rinsed and drained
- ✓ 1 Tbsp. freshly squeezed lemon juice

- ✓ 1 Tbsp. minced chives
- ✓ To taste, a pinch of sea salt

Directions:

14 teaspoons Heat the butter and oil in a wok over medium heat. Mix in the shrimp and peas. 5 to 7 minutes, or until shrimp are coral pink. Cook until the wild rice is thoroughly heated, then season with salt and butter. Place on a plate. Top with chives and lemon juice. Serve.

Nutrition:

- ✓ 510 calories
- ✓ Carbohydrates: 0g
- ✓ Fat: 0g
- ✓ 0g protein

38 Salad de Valencia

Time to Prepare: 10 minutes

Time to cook: 0 minutes

10 servings

Ingredients:

- ✓ 1 tsp. Kalamata olives in oil, pitted, lightly drained, halved, julienned
- ✓ 1 small Romaine lettuce head, rinsed, spun-dried, and cut into bite-sized pieces
- ✓ 12 julienned small shallots
- ✓ 1 tsp. Mustard Dijon
- ✓ 12 small satsuma or tangerine, only the pulp
- ✓ 1 tsp. vinegar made from white wine
- ✓ 1 tsp. olive oil extra virgin
- ✓ 1 pinch of minced fresh thyme
- ✓ 1 tsp sea salt
- ✓ To taste, a pinch of black pepper

Directions:

Combine the vinegar, oil, fresh thyme, salt, mustard, black pepper, and honey, if using, in a mixing bowl. Whisk until the dressing emulsifies slightly. In a salad bowl, combine the remaining salad ingredients. When ready to serve, drizzle with dressing. Serve right away with 1 slice of sugar-free sourdough bread or saltine crackers.

Nutrition:

- ✓ 238 calories
- ✓ Carbohydrates: 23g
- ✓ Fat: 15g

39 Stir-Fry Tenderloin with Red and Green Grapes

Time to Prepare: 15 minutes

Time to cook: 25 minutes

4 servings

Ingredients:

- ✓ 6 oz. medallion Trimmed pork tenderloin, membrane removed
- ✓ salt from the sea
- ✓ sesame seed oil
- ✓ Vinaigrette with grapes
- ✓ 14 cup quartered green grapes
- ✓ 14 cup quartered red grapes
- ✓ freshly cracked black peppercorns
- ✓ 1 tsp. Freshly squeezed apple cider vinegar

Directions:

To make the vinaigrette, combine all ingredients in a mixing bowl. Allow cooling before serving. Preheat the stovetop or electric grill for at least 3 minutes. Season the pork lightly with salt and sesame oil. Grill for 10 to 12 minutes or until both sides are well-seared. Take off the grill. Cover with aluminum foil and set aside for 5 minutes. Plate the cooked pork medallion. Finish with a vinaigrette. Serve.

Nutrition:

- ✓ 330 calories
- ✓ Carbohydrates: 28g
- ✓ Fat: 9g
- ✓ 27g protein

40 Eggs in Aioli

Time to prepare: 20 minutes

Time to cook: 0 minutes

12 servings

Ingredients:

- ✓ two egg yolks
- ✓ 1 garlic clove, grated

- ✓ 2 Tbsp. water
- ✓ 12 cup virgin olive oil
- ✓ 14 cups freshly squeezed lemon juice, pips removed
- ✓ ¼ tsp. salt from the sea
- ✓ 1 teaspoon cayenne pepper powder
- ✓ To taste, a pinch of white pepper

Directions:

Blend garlic, egg yolks, salt, and water until smooth. Slowly drizzle in the olive oil until the dressing emulsifies. Mix in the remaining ingredients. Adjust the seasoning to taste. Pour into an airtight container and store until needed.

Nutrition:

- ✓ 100 calories
- ✓ 1 gram of carbohydrates
- ✓ Fat: 11g
- ✓ 0g protein

41 Spaghetti Squash with Aioli

Time to Prepare: 10 minutes

Time to cook: 10 minutes

4 servings

Ingredients:

- ✓ 1 spaghetti squash, halved lengthwise and seeds removed
- ✓ 14 cups Aioli (eggs)
- ✓ drizzled with olive oil
- ✓ salt from the sea
- ✓ to taste, black pepper

Directions:

Heat the oven to 375°F/190°C. Grease the baking sheet lightly with oil using a pastry brush.Drizzle more oil over the cut sides of the squash and season liberally with salt and pepper.Place the vegetables, cut side down, on a baking sheet and roast for 40 to 45 minutes or until the squash is fork-tender.Remove and allow to cool. Turn the squash over and fork through the flesh to make spaghetti strands.In a mixing bowl, combine the veggie noodles and 14 cups of the aioli. Gently toss to combine. Taste and add more aioli if desired. Season with salt and pepper to taste; serve.

Nutrition:

- ✓ 31 calories
- ✓ Carbohydrates: 7g
- ✓ Fat: 1g

✓ 1g protein

42 Stew with Ginger Chicken

Time to Prepare: 10 minutes

Time to cook: 20 minutes

6 servings

Ingredients:

- ✓ 14 cups diced chicken thigh fillet
- ✓ 14 cups prepared egg noodles
- ✓ 1 peeled and diced unripe papaya
- ✓ 1 cup low-sodium, low-fat chicken broth
- ✓ 1 medallion peeled and crushed ginger
- ✓ a pinch of onion powder
- ✓ a pinch of garlic powder to taste
- ✓ 1 quart of water
- ✓ 1 tsp. sauce de Poisson
- ✓ a pinch of white pepper
- ✓ 1 piece minced small bird's eye chili

Directions:

Place all of the ingredients in a large Dutch oven over high heat. Boil.

Reduce the heat to the lowest setting. Replace the lid.Cook for 20 minutes or until the papaya is fork-tender. Turn off the heat. Consume on its own or with 12 cupsof cooked rice. Serve hot.

Nutrition:

- ✓ 273 calories
- ✓ Carbohydrates: 15g
- ✓ Fat: 9g
- ✓ 33g protein

43 Taro with Coconut Sauce

Time to Prepare: 10 minutes

Time to cook: 20 minutes

5 servings

Ingredients:
- ✓ 4 cups taro leaves, dried
- ✓ 2 coconut cream cans divided
- ✓ 14 cups 90% lean ground pork
- ✓ 1 tsp. prawn paste
- ✓ 1 minced bird's eye chili

Directions:

Except for 1 can of coconut cream, combine all ingredients in a crockpot set on medium heat. Close the lid. Cook for 3 to 312 hours, stirring occasionally.Before turning off the heat, add the remaining can of coconut cream. Serve with a stir.

Nutrition:

- ✓ 264 calories
- ✓ 8g carbs
- ✓ Fat: 24g
- ✓ 4g protein

44 Salmon Steak with Herbs de Provence

Time to Prepare: 10 minutes

Time to cook: 5 minutes

4 servings

Ingredients:

- ✓ 1 lb. 1/8 teaspoon cayenne pepper, rinsed salmon steak
- ✓ 1 teaspoon chili powder
- ✓ 12 teaspoon cumin
- ✓ 2 minced garlic cloves

✓ 1 tablespoon extra virgin olive oil

✓ 34 teaspoon salt

✓ 1 teaspoon black pepper, freshly ground

Directions:

Preheat the oven to 350 degrees Fahrenheit.Combine cayenne pepper, chili powder, cumin, salt, and black pepper in a mixing bowl. Place aside.Drizzle the salmon steak with olive oil. Rub both sides together. Rub the garlic and spice mixture together. Allow for a 10-minute resting period.Prepare an ovenproof skillet after the flavors have melded. Warm the olive oil. Season the salmon for 4 minutes on both sides once it is hot.Place the skillet in the oven. 10 minutes in the oven. Serve.

Nutrition:

✓ 210 calories

✓ Carbohydrates: 0g

✓ Fat: 14g

✓ 19g protein

45 Salad with Smoked Salmon

Time to Prepare: 15 minutes

Time to cook: 20 minutes

4 servings

Ingredients:

- ✓ 2 baby fennel bulbs, thinly sliced (reserve some fronds)
- ✓ 1 tablespoon rinsed and drained salted baby capers
- ✓ 12 cup plain yogurt
- ✓ 2 tablespoons chopped parsley

- ✓ 1 tablespoon freshly squeezed lemon juice
- ✓ 2 tablespoons chopped fresh chives
- ✓ 1 tablespoon fresh tarragon, chopped
- ✓ 180g low-salt sliced smoked salmon
- ✓ 12 thinly sliced red onion
- ✓ 1 teaspoon finely grated lemon rind
- ✓ 12 cups rinsed French green lentils
- ✓ 60g baby spinach, fresh
- ✓ 12 sliced avocado
- ✓ a smidgeon of caster sugar

Directions:

Fill a large saucepan halfway with water and boil over medium heat.

Once the water is boiling, cook the lentils for 20 minutes or until tender; drain well.Meanwhile, preheat a chargrill pan over high heat in advance. Spray the fennel slices with oil and cook for 2 minutes per side or until tender.In a food processor, combine the chives, parsley, yogurt, tarragon, lemon rind, and capers until completely smooth. Season with pepper to taste.In a large mixing bowl, combine the onion, sugar, juice, and a pinch of salt. Set aside for a few minutes before draining.In a large mixing bowl, combine the lentils, onion, fennel, avocado, and spinach. Divide the mixture evenly among the plates, then top with the fish. Sprinkle with the remaining fennel fronds and fresh parsley. Drizzle the green goddess dressing on top. Enjoy.

Nutrition:
- ✓ kcal: 368
- ✓ Fat: 14 g
- ✓ 8 g fiber
- ✓ 20 g protein

46 Couscous Pilaf with Turkey

Time to prepare: 20 minutes

Time to cook: 20 minutes

4 servings

Ingredients:

- ✓ 14-pound minced turkey
- ✓ 12 teaspoon cinnamon powder
- ✓ 1 finely chopped small red onion
- ✓ 14 tsp dried chili flakes
- ✓ 2 crushed garlic cloves
- ✓ 1 lemon, juiced; finely grated rind
- ✓ 12 teaspoon coriander powder
- ✓ 34 teaspoon ginger powder
- ✓ 1 cup fresh, tightly packed mint leaves
- ✓ 12 teaspoon cumin powder
- ✓ 1 couscous cup
- ✓ 12 cups dried cranberries
- ✓ 1 cup of hot water
- ✓ 2 tbsp toasted, chopped pistachios
- ✓ 1 cup fresh, tightly packed coriander leaves
- ✓ To serve, extra virgin olive oil

Directions:

In a skillet, heat the oil until it is hot. After that, add the onion and garlic and cook for 2 minutes, stirring frequently. Combine the ground coriander, cumin, ginger, chili, and cinnamon in a mixing bowl. Cook for another minute, frequently stirring to prevent burning, until aromatic. Turn the heat up to high and add the turkey. Cook for 6 minutes more or until thoroughly cooked and browned. Remember to break up the mince with a large wooden spoon as you cook the meat.Meanwhile, in a heatproof bowl, combine the cranberries, couscous, lemon juice, rind, and water. Cover with plastic wrap and set aside for 5 minutes to absorb before fluffing with a large fork. Season with pepper to taste.Half of the coriander and mint should be finely chopped. Toss the couscous with the turkey mixture, coriander, and mint. Combine thoroughly. Drizzle with more oil after sprinkling with pistachios.

Nutrition:

- ✓ kcal: 200
- ✓ Fat: 14 g
- ✓ 3 g fiber
- ✓ 34 g protein

47 Broccoli with anchovies and almonds

Time to Prepare: 10 minutes

Time to cook: 10 minutes

6 servings

Ingredients:

- ✓ 2 broccolini bunches, trimmed
- ✓ 1 tbsp olive oil (extra virgin)
- ✓ 1 fresh long red chili, deseeded and finely chopped
- ✓ 2 thinly sliced garlic cloves
- ✓ 14 cups coarsely chopped natural almonds
- ✓ 2 teaspoons finely grated lemon rind
- ✓ a squeeze of fresh lemon juice
- ✓ 4 chopped anchovies in oil

Directions:

In a large saucepan, heat the oil until it is hot. Stir in the anchovies, garlic, chili, and lemon rind. Cook for 30 seconds, frequently stirring, until aromatic. Cook for another minute, frequently stirring, after adding the almond. Remove from the heat and season with fresh lemon juice.The broccolini should then be placed in a steamer basket over a saucepan of simmering water. Cook, covered, until crisp-2 to 3 minutes, or until tender. Drain well before transferring to a large serving plate. Serve with the almond mixture on top. Enjoy.

Nutrition:

- ✓ kcal: 350
- ✓ Fat: 7 g
- ✓ 3 g fiber
- ✓ 6 g protein

48 Stuffed Peppers with Amaranth and Quinoa

Time to prepare: 20 minutes

1 hour and 10 minutes to cook

4 servings

Ingredients:

- ✓ 2 teaspoons amaranth
- ✓ 1 medium trimmed and grated zucchini
- ✓ 2 diced vine-ripened tomatoes
- ✓ 2/3 cup quinoa (approximately 135 g)
- ✓ 1 medium onion, finely chopped
- ✓ 2 garlic cloves, crushed
- ✓ 1 teaspoon cumin powder
- ✓ 2 tbsp sunflower seeds, lightly toasted
- ✓ 75g fresh ricotta cheese

- ✓ 2 teaspoons currants
- ✓ 4 large capsicums, halved lengthwise and seeded
- ✓ 2 tablespoons chopped flat-leaf parsley

Directions:

Line a baking tray, preferably large, with nonstick baking paper and preheat your oven to 350 F ahead of time. Fill a medium-sized saucepan halfway with water, add the amaranth and quinoa, and boil over medium heat. Reduce the heat to low, cover, and leave to simmer for 12 to 15 minutes or until the grains are al dente and the water has been absorbed. Set aside after removing from the heat.Meanwhile, lightly coat a large frying pan with oil and heat over medium heat. Once hot, add the onion and zucchini and cook for a few minutes, stirring, until softened. Cook for a minute after adding the cumin and garlic. Set aside to cool after removing from the heat.In a large mixing bowl, combine the grains, onion mixture, sunflower seeds, currants, parsley, ricotta, and tomato; give the ingredients a good stir until well combined—season with pepper and salt to taste.Fill the capsicums with the prepared quinoa mixture and arrange them on the baking sheet, covering them with aluminum foil. Bake for 17 to 20 minutes. Remove the foil and bake for 15 to 20 minutes more, or until the stuffing is golden and the vegetables are fork-tender.

Nutrition:

- ✓ kcal: 200
- ✓ Fat: 8.5 g
- ✓ 8 g fiber
- ✓ 15 g protein

49 Garlic and Parsley Dressed Grilled Ocean Trout

Time to prepare: 20 minutes

Time to cook: 25 minutes

8 servings

Ingredients:

- ✓ 12-pound fillet of trout, preferably ocean trout, boned and skin on
- ✓ 4 garlic cloves, thinly sliced
- ✓ 2 tablespoons coarsely chopped capers
- ✓ 12 cups fresh flat-leaf parsley
- ✓ 1 red chili, preferably long and thinly sliced
- ✓ 2 tbsp freshly squeezed lemon juice
- ✓ 12 cups extra virgin olive oil

✓ To serve lemon wedges

Directions:

Brush the trout with about 2 tablespoons of oil, ensuring that all sides are well coated. Preheat your grill over high heat, preferably with the hood closed. Reduce the heat to medium and place the coated trout on the grill plate, skin side up. CookFor a few minutes, until partially cooked and golden. Cook until the trout is cooked, 12 to 15 minutes, with the hood closed. Place the fillet on a large serving platter.

Meanwhile, heat the leftover oil; garlic in a small saucepan over low heat until just heated through; the garlic begins to change color. Remove the heat and stir in the capers, lemon juice, and chili. Drizzle the prepared dressing over the trout and top with fresh parsley leaves. Serve immediately with fresh lemon wedges, and enjoy.

Nutrition:

✓ kcal: 170
✓ Fat: 30 g
✓ 2 g fiber
✓ 37 grams of protein

50 Sandwich with Smashed Chickpea Avocado Salad and Cranberries

Time to Prepare: 10 minutes

Time to cook: 10 minutes

2 servings

Ingredients:

- ✓ 4 gluten-free bread slices
- ✓ 1 can rinse and drain chickpeas
- ✓ salt and black pepper
- ✓ 2 teaspoons freshly squeezed lemon juice
- ✓ 1 medium ripe avocado
- ✓ 14 cups dried cranberries
- ✓ Toppings: arugula, spinach, or red onion

Directions:

In a medium-sized mixing bowl, mash the chickpeas with a large fork. Add the avocado and mash again with the same fork until completely smooth; don't worry if it has some chunky pieces.Season with pepper and salt to taste after adding the cranberries and lemon juice. Refrigerate until ready to serve.To serve, toast the bread and spread about 12 of the chickpea avocado salad on one slice. Serve with arugula, spinach, or red onion on top. Top with another toasted piece and cut in half. Serve right away and enjoy.

Nutrition:

- ✓ kcal: 405
- ✓ Fat: 15 g
- ✓ 17 g fiber
- ✓ 12 g protein

51 delicious Tuna Salad

Time to Prepare: 10 minutes

Time to cook: 15 minutes

2 servings

Ingredients:

- ✓ 2 drained cans of tuna packed in water (5 oz each)
- ✓ 14 cups of mayonnaise
- ✓ 2 tbsp. fresh basil, chopped
- ✓ 1 tablespoon freshly squeezed lemon juice
- ✓ 2 tbsp. chopped fire-roasted red peppers
- ✓ 14 cups chopped kalamata or mixed olives
- ✓ 2 vine-ripened tomatoes, large
- ✓ 1 teaspoon capers

✓ 2 tablespoons minced red onion

✓ Season with pepper and salt to taste.

Directions:

In a large mixing bowl, combine all ingredients (except the tomatoes); give the ingredients a good stir until well combined. Cut the tomatoes into sixths and gently pry them open. Scoop the tuna salad mixture into the center; serve immediately and enjoy.

Nutrition:

✓ kcal: 405

✓ Fat: 24 g

✓ 3.2 g fiber

✓ 37 g protein

52 Chili with Turkey

Time to Prepare: 15 minutes

Time to cook: 4 hours and 10 minutes

8 servings

Ingredients:

✓ 1 pound ground turkey (ideally 99% lean)

- ✓ 2 cans of rinsed and drained red kidney beans (15 oz each)
- ✓ 1 chopped red pepper
- ✓ 2 tins tomato sauce (15 oz each)
- ✓ 1 jar (drained) deli-sliced tamed jalapeno peppers (16 oz)
- ✓ 2 cans diced petite tomatoes (15 oz each)
- ✓ 1 teaspoon cumin
- ✓ 1 small yellow pepper, chopped
- ✓ 2 cans of black beans, rinsed and drained (15 oz each)
- ✓ 1 cup frozen corn
- ✓ 2 teaspoon chili powder
- ✓ 1 tablespoon extra virgin olive oil
- ✓ To taste, black pepper and salt
- ✓ 1 medium diced onion
- ✓ Optional garnishes include green onions, avocado, shredded cheese, and Greek yogurt/sour cream.

Directions:

In a large skillet, heat the oil until it is hot. When finished, carefully place the turkey in the hot skillet and cook until brown. Fill the bottom of your slow cooker, preferably 6 quarts, with turkey.Combine the jalapenos, corn, peppers, onion, diced tomatoes, tomato sauce, beans, cumin, and chili powder in a mixing bowl. Mix, then season with pepper and salt to taste.Cook for 6 hours on low heat or 4 hours on high heat, covered. Serve with optional garnishes, and enjoy.

Nutrition:

- ✓ kcal: 455
- ✓ Fat: 9 g
- ✓ 19 g fiber
- ✓ 38 g protein

53 Wrapped Kale Caesar Salad with Grilled Chicken

Time to Prepare: 10 minutes

Time to cook: 20 minutes

2 servings

Ingredients:

- ✓ 6 cups curly kale, cut into bite-sized pieces
- ✓ 12 cooked coddled egg
- ✓ 8 ounces of thinly sliced grilled chicken
- ✓ 12 tsp Dijon mustard
- ✓ 34 cups finely shredded Parmesan cheese
- ✓ black pepper, ground
- ✓ salt kosher

- ✓ 1 minced garlic clove
- ✓ 1 cup quartered cherry tomatoes
- ✓ 1/8 cup freshly squeezed lemon juice
- ✓ 2 large tortillas or 2 flatbreads Lavash
- ✓ 1 teaspoon honey or agave
- ✓ 1/8 cup extra virgin olive oil

Directions:

Mix half of the coddled egg, mustard, minced garlic, honey, olive oil, and lemon juice in a large mixing bowl. Whisk until the mixture resembles dressing. Season to taste with pepper and salt.Toss in the cherry tomatoes, chicken, and kale until evenly coated with the dressing, then top with 14 cups of parmesan.Spread the flatbreads and evenly distribute the prepared salad on top of the wraps; sprinkle with 14 cups of parmesan.Roll the wraps up and cut them in half. Serve right away and enjoy.

Nutrition:

- ✓ kcal: 511
- ✓ Fat: 29 g
- ✓ 2.8 g fiber
- ✓ 50 g protein

54 Tilapia Baked with Pecan Rosemary Topping

Time to Prepare: 10 minutes

Time to cook: 20 minutes

4 servings

Ingredients:

- ✓ 4 fillets of tilapia (4 ounces each)
- ✓ 12 teaspoon brown sugar or palm sugar
- ✓ 2 teaspoons chopped fresh rosemary
- ✓ 1/3 cup chopped raw pecans
- ✓ Cayenne pepper, a pinch
- ✓ 12 tablespoon olive oil
- ✓ 1 big egg white
- ✓ a quarter teaspoon of salt
- ✓ 1/3 cup panko breadcrumbs (ideally whole wheat)

Directions:

Preheat your oven to 350°F.In a small baking dish, combine the pecans, breadcrumbs, coconut palm sugar, rosemary, cayenne pepper, and salt. Toss in the olive oil. Bake for 7–8 minutes until the mixture is light golden brown.Preheat the oven to 400°F and coat a large glass baking dish with cooking spray.In a shallow dish, whisk the egg white. In batches, dip the fish (one at a time) into the egg white, then lightly coat in the pecan mixture. In the baking dish, place the coated fillets.Apply the remaining pecan mixture to the tilapia fillets.Bake for 8 to 10 minutes. Serve right away and enjoy.

Nutrition:

- ✓ kcal: 222
- ✓ Fat: 10 g
- ✓ 2 g fiber
- ✓ 27 g protein

55 Egg Salad for Healthy Eating

Time to Prepare: 10 minutes

Time to cook: 0 minutes

2 servings

Ingredients:

- ✓ 6 hard-boiled organic pasture-raised eggs

- ✓ a single avocado

- ✓ 14 cups Greek yogurt
- ✓ 2 tablespoons mayonnaise made with olive oil
- ✓ 1 tablespoon fresh dill
- ✓ to taste, sea salt
- ✓ Serve with lettuce

Directions:

Combine the hard-boiled eggs and avocado.Combine the Greek yogurt, olive oil, mayonnaise, and fresh dill in a mixing bowl.Season with sea salt to taste. Serve on a lettuce bed.

Nutrition:

- ✓ Carbohydrates in total: 18g
- ✓ 10g dietary fiber
- ✓ 23g protein
- ✓ 38g total fat
- ✓ 486 calories

56 Fruit Salad in the Winter

Time to Prepare: 10 minutes

Time to cook: 0 minutes

6 servings

Ingredients:

- ✓ 4 cubed cooked sweet potatoes (1-inch cubes)
- ✓ 3 cubed pears (1-inch cubes)
- ✓ 1 cup halved grapes
- ✓ 1 cubed apple
- ✓ 12 cup pecan halves
- ✓ 2 teaspoons olive oil
- ✓ 1 teaspoon red wine vinegar
- ✓ 2 teaspoons raw honey

Directions:

Whisk together the olive oil, red wine vinegar, and raw honey to make the dressing. Set aside.Divide the chopped fruit, sweet potato, and pecan halves among six serving bowls. Drizzle the dressing over each bowl.

Nutrition:

- ✓ Carbohydrates (total): 40g

✓ 6g dietary fiber

✓ 3g protein

✓ 11g total fat

✓ 251 calories

57 Salad with Salmon Made Simple

Time to Prepare: 10 minutes

Time to cook: 0 minutes

1 serving

Ingredients:

✓ 1 cup arugula, organic

✓ 1 wild-caught salmon can

✓ 12 avocados (sliced)

✓ 1 teaspoon of olive oil

✓ 1 tablespoon Dijon mustard

✓ 1 tablespoon sea salt

Directions:

To make the dressing, mix the olive oil, Dijon mustard, and sea salt in a mixing bowl. Place aside.Assemble the salad with the arugula as the base and the salmon and avocado slices on top.Drizzle the dressing on top.

Nutrition:

- ✓ Carbohydrates in total: 7g
- ✓ 5g dietary fiber
- ✓ 48g protein
- ✓ 37g total fat
- ✓ 553 calories

58 Salad with Pasta

Time to Prepare: 15 minutes

Time to cook: 10 minutes

6 servings

Ingredients:

- ✓ 1 pound gluten-free fusilli pasta
- ✓ 1 cup sliced grape tomatoes
- ✓ 1 bunch of chopped fresh cilantro
- ✓ 1 cup halved olives

- ✓ 1 cup chopped fresh basil
- ✓ 12 cup olive oil
- ✓ to taste, sea salt

Directions:

Combine the olive oil, basil, cilantro, and sea salt in a mixing bowl. Place aside.Cook the pasta according to the package instructions, then drain and rinse.Combine the pasta, tomatoes, and olives in a mixing bowl.Toss in the olive oil mixture until well combined.

Nutrition:

- ✓ Carbohydrates (total): 66g
- ✓ 5g dietary fiber
- ✓ 13g protein
- ✓ 23g total fat
- ✓ 525 calories

59 Salad with Spinach and Beans

Time to Prepare: 10 minutes

Time to cook: 5 minutes

1 serving

Ingredients:

- ✓ 1 cup spinach, fresh
- ✓ 14 cups black beans, canned
- ✓ 12 cups garbanzo beans, canned
- ✓ 12 cup cremini mushroom
- ✓ 2 tbsp balsamic vinaigrette (organic)
- ✓ 1 teaspoon of olive oil

Directions:

Cook the cremini mushrooms in the olive oil for 5 minutes over low to medium heat until lightly browned.To make the salad, place the fresh spinach on a plate and top it with the beans, mushrooms, and balsamic vinaigrette.

Nutrition:

- ✓ Carbohydrates in total: 26g
- ✓ 8g dietary fiber
- ✓ 9g protein
- ✓ 15g total fat
- ✓ 274 calories

60 Salad with Kale

Time to Prepare: 10 minutes

Time to cook: 0 minutes

1 serving

Ingredients:

- ✓ 1 cup kale, fresh
- ✓ 12 cup blueberries
- ✓ 12 cups pitted and halved cherries
- ✓ 14 cups cranberries, dried
- ✓ 1 teaspoon sesame seeds
- ✓ 2 teaspoons olive oil
- ✓ 1 lemon juice

Directions:

Toss the kale into the dressing after combining the olive oil and lemon juice.Toss the kale leaves with the fresh blueberries, cherries, and cranberries in a salad bowl.Sesame seeds should be sprinkled on top.

Nutrition:

- ✓ Carbohydrates (total): 48g

- ✓ 7g dietary fiber

- ✓ 6g protein

- ✓ 33g total fat

- ✓ 477 calories

CHAPTER 05: DINNER RECIPE

61 Vegetables Roasted with Sweet Potatoes and White Beans

Time to Prepare: 15 minutes

Time to cook: 25 minutes

4 servings

Ingredients:

- ✓ 2 small diced sweet potatoes
- ✓ 12 red onions, diced into 14-inch cubes
- ✓ 1 medium peeled and thinly sliced carrot
- ✓ 4 ounces trimmed green beans
- ✓ 14 cup virgin olive oil
- ✓ 1 teaspoon sea salt
- ✓ 14 teaspoons black pepper, freshly ground
- ✓ 1 can (1512 oz.) white beans, drained and rinsed
- ✓ 1 tablespoon lemon zest, minced or grated
- ✓ 1 tablespoon fresh dill, chopped

Directions:

Preheat the oven to 400 degrees Fahrenheit. On a large-rimmed baking sheet, combine the sweet potatoes, onion, carrot, green beans, oil, salt, and pepper. Arrange everything in a single layer. Cook for 20 to 25 minutes or until the vegetables are tender. Mix in the white beans, lemon zest, and dill before serving.

Nutrition:

- ✓ 315 calories
- ✓ 13g total fat
- ✓ 42g total carbohydrates
- ✓ 5g sugar
- ✓ 13g fiber
- ✓ 10g protein
- ✓ 632mg sodium

62 Greens and roasted tofu

Time to Prepare: 10 minutes

Time to cook: 20 minutes

4 servings

Ingredients:

- ✓ 3 cups kale or baby spinach
- ✓ 1 tbsp sesame seed oil
- ✓ 1 tablespoon minced ginger
- ✓ 1 minced garlic clove
- ✓ 1 pound firm tofu, diced into 1-inch cubes
- ✓ 1 tablespoon gluten-free soy sauce or tamari
- ✓ 14 tsp red pepper flakes (optional)
- ✓ 1 tsp. rice vinegar
- ✓ 2 thinly sliced scallions

Directions:

Preheat the oven to 400 degrees Fahrenheit. Combine the spinach, oil, ginger, and garlic on a large-rimmed baking sheet. Bake for 3 to 5 minutes or until the spinach has wilted. Toss in the tofu, tamari, and red pepper flakes (if using) until well combined. Bake for 10 to 15 minutes or until the tofu begins to brown. Serve with the vinegar and scallions on top.

Nutrition:

- ✓ 121 calories
- ✓ 8g total fat
- ✓ 4g total carbohydrates

- ✓ 1 gram sugar
- ✓ 2g fiber
- ✓ 10g protein
- ✓ 258mg sodium

63 Summer Vegetables with Italian Seasoning and Tofu

Time to Prepare: 10 minutes

Time to cook: 20 minutes

4 servings

Ingredients:

- ✓ 2 large zucchinis, 14-inch slices
- ✓ 2 large summer squash, sliced 14-inch thick
- ✓ 1 pound firm tofu, diced into 1-inch cubes
- ✓ 1 cup water or vegetable broth
- ✓ 3 tbsp extra virgin olive oil
- ✓ 2 sliced garlic cloves
- ✓ 1 teaspoon sea salt
- ✓ 1 tsp Italian herb seasoning mix
- ✓ 14 teaspoons black pepper, freshly ground

Directions:

Preheat the oven to 400 degrees Fahrenheit. Combine the zucchini, squash, tofu, broth, oil, garlic, salt, Italian herb seasoning blend, and pepper on a large-rimmed baking sheet. Roast for 20 minutes. Serve with the basil on top.

Nutrition:
- ✓ 213 calories
- ✓ 16g total fat
- ✓ 9g total carbohydrate
- ✓ 4g sugar
- ✓ 3g fiber
- ✓ 13g protein
- ✓ 806mg sodium

64 Broccoli, Cauliflower, and Tofu with Red Onion Spice

Time to Prepare: 10 minutes

Time to cook: 25 minutes

2 servings

Ingredients:

- ✓ 2 cups florets broccoli
- ✓ 2 cups florets cauliflower
- ✓ 1 medium diced red onion
- ✓ 3 tbsp extra virgin olive oil
- ✓ 1 teaspoon sea salt
- ✓ 14 teaspoons black pepper, freshly ground
- ✓ 1 pound firm tofu, diced into 1-inch cubes
- ✓ 1 minced garlic clove
- ✓ 1 14-inch pieces minced fresh ginger

Directions:

Preheat the oven to 400 degrees Fahrenheit. On a largerimmed baking sheet, toss the broccoli, cauliflower, onion, oil, salt, and pepper Roast for 10 to 15 minutes or until the vegetables are softened. Combine the tofu, garlic, and ginger in a mixing bowl. Roast for 10 minutes. Mix the ingredients on the baking sheet gently to combine the tofu and vegetables, then serve.

Nutrition:

- ✓ 210 calories
- ✓ 15g total fat
- ✓ 11g total carbohydrates

- ✓ 4g sugar
- ✓ 4g fiber
- ✓ 12g protein
- ✓ 626mg sodium

65 Baked Tempeh and Root Vegetables

Time to Prepare: 10 minutes

Time to cook: 30 minutes

4 servings

Ingredients:

- ✓ 1 tbsp olive oil (extra virgin)
- ✓ 1 large diced sweet potato
- ✓ 2 thinly sliced carrots
- ✓ 1 fennel bulb, trimmed and diced 14 inches
- ✓ 2 teaspoons fresh ginger, minced
- ✓ 1 minced garlic clove
- ✓ 12 ounces tempeh, diced into 12-inch cubes
- ✓ 12 cup veggie broth

- ✓ 1 tablespoon gluten-free soy sauce or tamari
- ✓ 2 thinly sliced scallions

Directions:

Preheat the oven to 400 degrees Fahrenheit. Using the oil, grease a baking sheet. Arrange the sweet potato, carrots, fennel, ginger, and garlic on a baking sheet in a single layer. Bake for 15 minutes or until the vegetables have softened. Combine the tempeh, broth, and tamari in a mixing bowl. Bake for 10 to 15 minutes or until the tempeh is heated and lightly browned. Stir in the scallions and serve.

Nutrition:

- ✓ 276 calories
- ✓ 13g total fat
- ✓ 26g total carbohydrate
- ✓ 5g sugar
- ✓ 4g fiber
- ✓ 19g protein
- ✓ 397mg sodium

66 Chicken with Garlic and Vegetables

Time to Prepare: 10 minutes

Time to cook: 45 minutes

4 servings

Ingredients:

- ✓ 2 tsp extra virgin olive oil
- ✓ 1 leek, only the white part, thinly sliced
- ✓ 2 large zucchinis, 14-inch slices
- ✓ 4 chicken breasts, bone-in, and skin-on
- ✓ 3 minced garlic cloves
- ✓ 1 teaspoon sea salt
- ✓ 1 tsp. dried oregano
- ✓ 14 teaspoons black pepper, freshly ground
- ✓ 12 glasses of white wine
- ✓ 1 lemon juice

Directions:

Preheat the oven to 400 degrees Fahrenheit. Brush the baking sheet with oil. Place the zucchini and leeks on a baking sheet. Sprinkle the garlic, salt, oregano, and pepper over the chicken, skin-side up. Pour in the wine. Cook for 35 to 40 minutes. Remove and set aside for 5 minutes to rest. Serve with lemon juice.

Nutrition:

- ✓ 315 calories

✓ 8g total fat

✓ 12g total carbohydrates

✓ 4g sugar

✓ 2g fiber

✓ 44g protein

✓ 685mg sodium

67 Chicken with Turmeric-Spiced Sweet Potatoes, Apple, and Onion

Time to Prepare: 15 minutes

Time to cook: 45 minutes

4 servings

Ingredients:

✓ 2 tablespoons room temperature unsalted butter

✓ 2 large sweet potatoes

✓ 1 Granny Smith apple, large

✓ 1 medium thinly sliced onion

✓ 4 chicken breasts, bone-in, and skin-on

✓ 1 teaspoon sea salt

✓ 1 tablespoon turmeric

✓ 1 tsp. dried sage

✓ 14 teaspoons black pepper, freshly ground

✓ 1 cup white wine, apple cider, or chicken broth

Directions:

Preheat the oven to 400 degrees Fahrenheit. Using the butter, grease a baking sheet. Arrange the sweet potatoes, apple, and onion on a baking sheet in a single layer. Season the chicken with salt, turmeric, sage, pepper, and skin side up. Pour in the cider. Cook for 35 to 40 minutes. Remove from the oven, set aside for 5 minutes, and serve.

Nutrition:

✓ 386 calories

✓ 12g total fat

✓ 26g total carbohydrate

✓ 10g sugar

✓ 4g fiber

✓ 44g protein

✓ 932mg sodium

68 Carrots with honey-roasted chicken thighs

Time to Prepare: 10 minutes

Time to cook: 50 minutes

4 servings

Ingredients:

- ✓ 2 tablespoons room temperature unsalted butter
- ✓ 3 thinly sliced large carrots
- ✓ 2 minced garlic cloves
- ✓ 4 chicken thighs, bone-in, and skin-on
- ✓ 1 teaspoon sea salt
- ✓ 12 tsp dried rosemary
- ✓ 14 teaspoons black pepper, freshly ground
- ✓ 2 teaspoons honey
- ✓ 1 cup broth (chicken or vegetable)
- ✓ For serving, lemon wedges

Directions:

Preheat the oven to 400 degrees Fahrenheit. Using the butter, grease a baking sheet. Arrange the carrots and garlic on a baking sheet in a single layer. Season the chicken with salt, rosemary, and pepper and arrange it on top of the vegetables. Place the honey on top, followed by the broth. Cook for 40 to 45 minutes. Remove from the oven, set aside for 5 minutes, and serve with lemon wedges.

Nutrition:

- ✓ 428 calories
- ✓ 28g total fat
- ✓ Carbohydrates in total: 15g
- ✓ 11g sugar
- ✓ 2g fiber
- ✓ 30g protein
- ✓ 732mg sodium

69 Baked Sesame-Tamari Chicken with Green Beans

Time to Prepare: 10 minutes

Time to cook: 45 minutes

4 servings

Ingredients:

- ✓ 1 pound trimmed green beans
- ✓ 4 chicken breasts, bone-in, and skin-on
- ✓ 2 teaspoons honey
- ✓ 1 tbsp sesame seed oil
- ✓ 1 tablespoon gluten-free soy sauce or tamari

✓ 1 cup broth (chicken or vegetable)

Directions:

Preheat the oven to 400 degrees Fahrenheit. Arrange the green beans on a large baking sheet with a rim. Place the chicken on top of the beans, skin side up. Drizzle the honey, oil, and tamari over the top. Pour in the broth. Cook for 35 to 40 minutes. Remove from the oven, set aside for 5 minutes, and serve.

Nutrition:

✓ 378 calories
✓ 10g total fat
✓ 19g total carbohydrates
✓ 10g sugar
✓ 4g fiber
✓ 54g protein
✓ 336mg sodium

70 Turkey Breasts on a Sheet Pan with Golden Vegetables

Time to Prepare: 15 minutes

Time to cook: 45 minutes

4 servings

Ingredients:

- ✓ 2 tablespoons room temperature unsalted butter
- ✓ 1 medium-seeded and thinly sliced acorn squash
- ✓ 2 large peeled and thinly sliced golden beets
- ✓ 12 thinly sliced medium yellow onion
- ✓ 12 boneless skinless turkey breasts (1 to 2 pounds)
- ✓ 2 teaspoons honey
- ✓ 1 teaspoon sea salt
- ✓ 1 tablespoon turmeric
- ✓ 14 teaspoons black pepper, freshly ground
- ✓ 1 cup broth (chicken or vegetable)

Directions:

Preheat the oven to 400 degrees Fahrenheit. Using the butter, grease a baking sheet. Arrange the squash, beets, and onion on a baking sheet in a single layer. Place the turkey skin-side up on a plate. Drizzle the honey on top. Add the broth and season with salt, turmeric, and pepper. 35 to 45 minutes, or until an instant-read thermometer reads 165°F in the center of the turkey. Remove and set aside for 5 minutes to rest. Cut into slices and serve.

Nutrition:

- ✓ 383 calories
- ✓ 15g total fat
- ✓ Carbohydrates (total): 25g
- ✓ 13g sugar
- ✓ 3g fiber
- ✓ 37g protein
- ✓ 748mg sodium

71Steak on a Sheet Pan with Brussels Sprouts and Red Wine

Time to Prepare: 10 minutes

Time to cook: 20 minutes

4 servings

Ingredients:

- ✓ a pound of rib-eye steak
- ✓ 1 teaspoon sea salt
- ✓ 14 teaspoons black pepper, freshly ground
- ✓ 1 tbsp. unsalted butter

- ✓ 12 minced red onion
- ✓ 8 ounces trimmed and quartered Brussels sprouts
- ✓ 1-quart red wine
- ✓ 12 lemon juice

Directions:

Preheat the broiler to high heat.Season the steak with salt and pepper on a large-rimmed baking sheet. Broil for 2 to 3 minutes per side or until browned.Please turn off the oven and preheat it to 400°F.Place the steak on one side of a baking sheet and the butter, onion, Brussels sprouts, and wine on the other.Roast for 8 minutes. Remove and set aside for 5 minutes to rest.Serve with a squeeze of lemon juice.

Nutrition:

- ✓ 416 calories
- ✓ 27g total fat
- ✓ 8g total carbohydrate
- ✓ 2g sugar
- ✓ 3g fiber
- ✓ 22g protein
- ✓ 636mg sodium

72 Green Beans and Miso Salmon

Time to Prepare: 10 minutes

Time to cook: 25 minutes

4 servings

Ingredients:

- ✓ 1 tbsp sesame seed oil
- ✓ 1 pound trimmed green beans
- ✓ 1 pound salmon fillets, skin on, cut into 4 steaks
- ✓ 14 cup miso white
- ✓ 2 teaspoons gluten-free soy sauce or tamari
- ✓ 2 thinly sliced scallions

Directions:

Preheat the oven to 400 degrees Fahrenheit. Brush the baking sheet with oil.Place the green beans on the bottom, then the salmon on top, and brush each piece with miso.Cook for 20 to 25 minutes.Drizzle with tamari and sprinkle with scallions before serving.

Nutrition:

- ✓ 213 calories

- ✓ 7g total fat
- ✓ 13g total carbohydrates
- ✓ 3g sugar
- ✓ 5g fiber
- ✓ 27g protein
- ✓ 989mg sodium

73 Tilapia and Asparagus with Acorn Squash

Time to Prepare: 15 minutes

Time to cook: 30 minutes

4 servings

Ingredients:

- ✓ 2 tbsp extra virgin olive oil
- ✓ 1 medium acorn squash, seeded and sliced thinly or cut into wedges
- ✓ 1-pound asparagus, cut into 2-inch pieces after trimming the woody ends
- ✓ 1 large, thinly sliced shallot
- ✓ 1 pound fillets of tilapia

- ✓ 12 glasses of white wine
- ✓ 1 tablespoon fresh flat-leaf parsley, chopped
- ✓ 1 teaspoon sea salt
- ✓ 14 teaspoons black pepper, freshly ground

Directions:

Preheat the oven to 400 degrees Fahrenheit. Brush the baking sheet with oil.Arrange the squash, asparagus, and shallot on a baking sheet in a single layer. Roast for 8 to 10 minutes.Pour the wine over the tilapia.Season with parsley, salt, and pepper.Roast for 15 minutes. Remove and set aside for 5 minutes before serving.

Nutrition:

- ✓ 246 calories
- ✓ 8g total fat
- ✓ Carbohydrates (total): 17g
- ✓ 2g sugar
- ✓ 4g fiber
- ✓ 25g protein
- ✓ 639mg sodium

74 Baked Shrimp-Lime Zucchini and Corn

Time to Prepare: 10 minutes

Time to cook: 20 minutes

4 servings

Ingredients:

- ✓ 1 tbsp olive oil (extra virgin)
- ✓ 2 small zucchinis, diced into 14-inch cubes
- ✓ 1 frozen cup of corn kernels
- ✓ 2 thinly sliced scallions
- ✓ 1 teaspoon sea salt
- ✓ 12 teaspoon cumin powder
- ✓ 12 tsp chipotle chili powder
- ✓ 1 pound peeled shrimp (thawed if needed)
- ✓ 1 tablespoon fresh cilantro, finely chopped
- ✓ 1 lime zest and juice

Directions:

Preheat the oven to 400 degrees Fahrenheit. Brush the baking sheet with oil.Combine the zucchini, corn, scallions, salt, cumin, and chile powder on a baking sheet and mix well. Arrange everything in a single layer.Top with the shrimp. Cook for 15 to 20 minutes.Stir in the cilantro, lime zest, and juice before serving.

Nutrition:

- ✓ 184 calories
- ✓ 5g total fat
- ✓ 11g total carbohydrates
- ✓ 3g sugar
- ✓ 2g fiber
- ✓ 26g protein
- ✓ 846mg sodium

75 Broccoli and Almonds

Time to Prepare: 15 minutes

Time to cook: 5 minutes

6 servings

Ingredients:

- ✓ 1 deseeded and finely chopped fresh red chili
- ✓ 2 broccolini bunches, trimmed
- ✓ 1 tbsp olive oil (extra virgin)
- ✓ 2 thinly sliced garlic cloves
- ✓ 1/4 cup coarsely chopped natural almonds

✓ 2 teaspoons finely grated lemon rind

✓ 4 chopped anchovies in oil

✓ a squeeze of freshly squeezed lemon juice

Directions:

Preheat some oil in a skillet. 2 teaspoons lemon rind, anchovies, finely chopped chili, gloves, thinly sliced. Cook for about 30 seconds, stirring constantly.Cook for a minute after adding 1/4 cup of coarsely chopped almonds. Turn off the heat and sprinkle with lemon juice.Set the steamer basket over a saucepan of simmering water. Cover the broccolini in a basket.Cook for 3-4 minutes or until tender-crisp. Transfer to a serving platter after draining.Enjoy with the almond mixture on top!

Nutrition:

✓ 414 kilocalories

✓ 6.6 g fat

✓ 1.6 g total carbohydrates

✓ Protein content: 5.4 g

76 Tilapia with Rosemary Pecan Topping

Time to Prepare: 15 minutes

Time to cook: 18 minutes

4 servings

Ingredients:

- ✓ 4 fillets of tilapia
- ✓ 1/3 cup chopped raw pecans
- ✓ 1 white egg
- ✓ 1/3 cup panko breadcrumbs (whole wheat)
- ✓ 1 tablespoon brown sugar
- ✓ 12 teaspoon olive oil
- ✓ 2 teaspoons chopped fresh rosemary
- ✓ a quarter teaspoon of salt
- ✓ 1 tsp cayenne pepper

Directions:

In a baking dish, combine brown sugar, 1/3 cup breadcrumbs, 2 teaspoons fresh rosemary, a pinch of cayenne pepper, 1/8 teaspoon salt, and 1/3 cup chopped pecans. Combine everything.Drizzle with oil and toss until well coated—Preheat oven to 350°F.Bake for about 7-8 minutes or until golden brown. Raise the temperature to 400 degrees Fahrenheit.Spray the baking dish with nonstick cooking spray. Whisk the egg whites in a shallow dish, dip each fish fillet into the egg, and coat with the pecan mixture.Place the coated fillets in a baking dish, followed by the remaining pecan mixture.Bake for about 10 minutes or until thoroughly cooked. Serve immediately!

Nutrition:

- ✓ 222 kilocalories
- ✓ 10.8 g fat
- ✓ 6.7 g total carbohydrates
- ✓ Protein: 26.8 g

77 Trout Steamed with Red Bean and Chili Salsa

Time to Prepare: 15 minutes

Time to cook: 16 minutes

1 serving

Ingredients:

- ✓ 4 12 oz halved cherry tomatoes
- ✓ 1/4 unpeeled avocado
- ✓ Ocean trout fillet, 6 oz., skinless
- ✓ Serve with coriander leaves
- ✓ 2 tbsp. olive oil

- ✓ To serve lime wedges
- ✓ 4 12 oz rinsed and drained canned red kidney beans
- ✓ 1/2 thinly sliced red onion
- ✓ 1 tablespoon drained pickled jalapenos
- ✓ 1/2 teaspoon cumin powder
- ✓ 4 green olives from Sicily

Directions:

Place a steamer basket on top of a pot of simmering water. Cook for 10-12 minutes after adding the fish to the basket.Remove the fish and set it aside for a few minutes to rest. Meanwhile, heat some oil in a skillet.In a mixing bowl, combine pickled jalapenos, red kidney beans, olives, 1/2 teaspoon of cumin, and cherry tomatoes. Cook for 4-5 minutes, stirring constantly.Place the bean batter on a serving platter, then the trout. On top, sprinkle with coriander and onion.Serve with lime wedges and avocado slices. Steamed ocean trout with red bean and chili salsa isdelicious!

Nutrition:

- ✓ 243 kilocalories
- ✓ 33.2 g fat
- ✓ 18.8 g total carbohydrates
- ✓ Protein content: 44 g

78 Ratatouille

Time to Prepare: 15 minutes

Time to cook: 55 minutes

4 servings

Ingredients:
- ✓ 1 thickly sliced red onion
- ✓ 5 tbsp of olive oil
- ✓ 2 tbsp fresh thyme leaves
- ✓ 2 smashed garlic cloves
- ✓ 3 thickly sliced tomatoes
- ✓ 2 oregano sprigs
- ✓ 2 red bell peppers, cut in half and sides removed
- ✓ 1 cup pureed/sauced tomatoes
- ✓ 2 thickly sliced medium zucchini
- ✓ 1 thickly sliced small eggplant
- ✓ 2 thickly sliced medium summer squash
- ✓ Season with salt to taste.
- ✓ To taste, freshly ground black pepper

Directions:

Preheat the oven to 375 degrees Fahrenheit.A baking dish should be placed on a baking sheet in a small pot over medium heat and some olive oil. Cook for 1 minute or until garlic is fragrant.Turn off the heat and add 2 oregano sprigs. Allow it to rest for 15-20 minutes.Remove the oregano and garlic, and grease the baking dish with 2 tablespoons of oil.Spread 4 tablespoons of tomato puree evenly in the baking dish. Layer zucchini, eggplant, tomato, onion, and summer squash on top. Repeat the layering process.Brush the top with the remaining tomato puree. Drizzle with olive oil and season with pepper, salt, and thyme.Bake for 25-30 minutes or until the potatoes are tender. Allow cooling for 5-10 minutes. Serve immediately!

Nutrition:

- ✓ 283 kilocalories
- ✓ 18 g fat
- ✓ 30 g total carbohydrates
- ✓ 6 g of protein

79 Stuffed Italian Peppers

Time to Prepare: 15 minutes

Time to cook: 40 minutes

6 servings

Ingredients:

- ✓ 1 tsp. garlic powder
- ✓ 1/2 cup shredded mozzarella
- ✓ 1 lb. ground beef that is lean
- ✓ 1/2 cup grated parmesan cheese
- ✓ 3 bell peppers, cut lengthwise in half, stems, seeds, and ribs removed
- ✓ 1 package (10 oz.) of frozen spinach
- ✓ 2 cups tomato sauce
- ✓ 1 teaspoon of salt
- ✓ 1 tablespoon of Italian seasoning

Directions:

Coat a baking sheet with foil with nonstick spray. Place the peppers on a baking sheet.Cook the turkey in a nonstick skillet over medium heat until it is no longer pink.Cook for 8-10 minutes after adding 2 cups of marinara sauce and seasonings.Mix in the spinach and 1/2 cup of parmesan cheese. Stir until thoroughly combined.Preheat the oven to 450°F and spoon half a cup of the meat mixture into each pepper.Bake the peppers for 25-30 minutes. Allow cooling before serving.

Nutrition:

- ✓ 150 kilocalories
- ✓ 2 g fat
- ✓ 11 g total carbohydrates
- ✓ protein (20 g)

80 Salmon with Lemon Herbs and Zucchini

Time to Prepare: 15 minutes

Time to cook: 20 minutes

4 servings

Ingredients:

- ✓ 4 chopped zucchini
- ✓ 2 tbsp of olive oil
- ✓ Season with salt to taste.
- ✓ To taste, freshly ground black pepper

Regarding the Salmon:

- ✓ 4 fillets of salmon
- ✓ a half teaspoon of dried oregano
- ✓ 2 tablespoons chopped fresh parsley
- ✓ 2 tbsp. brown sugar, packed
- ✓ 2 tbsp lemon juice, freshly squeezed
- ✓ To taste kosher salt
- ✓ To taste, freshly ground black pepper
- ✓ 1 tbsp. Dijon mustard
- ✓ 1 tablespoon dried rosemary
- ✓ 2 minced garlic cloves
- ✓ 1 tablespoon dried thyme
- ✓ a half teaspoon of dried dill

Directions:

Spray the baking sheet with nonstick cooking spray. Preheat the oven to 400 degrees Fahrenheit.In a mixing bowl, combine the garlic, 1/2 teaspoon dried dill, 1 tablespoon Dijon mustard, 1/2 teaspoon dried oregano, 2 tablespoons brown sugar, lemon juice, 2 pinches thyme, and rosemary. Whisk until smooth, then season with pepper and salt to taste. Set it aside. Place the zucchini on a baking sheet sprayed with cooking spray. Drizzle with olive oil and season with pepper and salt. Arrange the salmon on top in an even layer and brush with the herb mixture.Bake for 18 minutes. Serve the lemon herb salmon and zucchini with parsley right away!

Nutrition:

- ✓ 330 kilocalories
- ✓ 16.7 g fat
- ✓ 14.7 g total carbohydrates
- ✓ Protein content: 31 g

81 Burgers with Sweet Potato and Black Beans

Time to Prepare: 15 minutes

Time to cook: 10 minutes

6 servings

Ingredients:

- ✓ 1/2 seeded and diced jalapeno
- ✓ 1 quinoa cup
- ✓ 6 hamburger buns (whole grain)
- ✓ 1 can of rinsed and drained black beans

✓ Cooking olive oil/coconut oil

✓ 1 medium sweet potato

✓ 1/2 cup diced red onion

✓ 4 tbsp oat flour (gluten-free)

✓ 2 minced garlic cloves

✓ 2 teaspoons cajun spicy seasoning

✓ 1/2 cup chopped cilantro

✓ 1 tablespoon cumin

✓ Sprouts

✓ Season with salt to taste.

✓ To taste, pepper

For the Cremation:

✓ 2 tablespoons chopped cilantro

✓ 1/2 avocado (diced)

✓ 4 tbsp low-fat sour cream or plain Greek yogurt

✓ 1 tsp. lime juice

Directions:

Rinse the quinoa with cold running water. Warm up a cup of water in a saucepan. Bring the quinoa to a boil.Cover and cook over low heat for about 15 minutes or until all the water hasbeen absorbed.Turn off the heat and fluff the quinoa with a fork. Then, transfer the quinoa to a bowl and set aside 5-10 minutes to cool.Poke the potato with a fork and microwave for a few minutes or until it is thoroughly cooked and soft. After cooking, peel the potato and set it aside to cool.In a food processor, combine 1 can of black beans, 12 cups chopped cilantro, 2 teaspoons Cajun seasoning, 12 cups diced onion, 1 teaspoon cumin, and 2 minced garlic cloves. Pulse until the mixture is smooth. Transfer to a bowl and top with cooked quinoa.Mix in the oat flour/bran. Make 6 patties out of the mixture. Refrigerate patties for about 30 minutes on a baking sheet.In a food processor, combine all of the Crema ingredients. Blend until smooth. Refrigerate after adjusting the salt to taste.Heat an oil-splattered skillet over medium heat. Cook each side of the patties for 3-4 minutes or until lightly golden. Serve with crema, sprouts, buns, and other toppings of your choice.

Nutrition:

- ✓ 206 kilocalories
- ✓ 6 g fat
- ✓ 33.9 g total carbohydrates
- ✓ Protein content: 7.9 g

82 Stuffed Peppers with Turkey and Quinoa

Time to Prepare: 15 minutes

Time to cook: 45 minutes

4 servings

Ingredients:

- ✓ 1 cup chopped fresh spinach
- ✓ 1 cup cooked quinoa
- ✓ 3 large yellow peppers, remove stems and seeds, cut in half
- ✓ 1 cup chicken stock
- ✓ 1.25 lb. ground turkey that is extra lean
- ✓ 1 cup tomato sauce (18 oz. can)
- ✓ 1 cup diced mushrooms
- ✓ 2 teaspoons minced garlic
- ✓ 1/4 cup diced sweet onion

Directions:

Preheat some oil in a skillet and add the vegetables. After about 5 minutes, add 2 teaspoons of minced garlic and the ground turkey. Cook until the meat is completely cooked. 1 cup of chicken broth and 1 cup of tomato sauce. Cook on low heat.Meanwhile, spray a baking pan with cooking spray. Place the bell peppers in the pan.When the quinoa is done, add it to the pan with the vegetables and turkey. Stir until thoroughly combined.Fill the bell peppers with the mixture. Preheat the oven to 400°F. Pour the remaining chicken broth into the baking pan around the peppers.Cook for about 30-35 minutes, covered with foil. Serve and have fun!

Nutrition:

- ✓ 640 kilocalories
- ✓ 13 g fat
- ✓ 74 g total carbohydrates
- ✓ Protein content: 53 g

83 Zoodles with Avocado Pesto and Salmon

Time to Prepare: 15 minutes

Time to cook: 25 minutes

4 servings

Ingredients:

- ✓ 1 teaspoon pesto
- ✓ 1 lemon
- ✓ 2 salmon steaks (frozen or fresh)
- ✓ 1 large spiralized zucchini

- ✓ 1 tablespoon ground black pepper
- ✓ a single avocado
- ✓ 1/4 cup grated parmesan
- ✓ Seasoning from Italy

Directions:

Preheat the oven to 375°F. Bake for 20 minutes, seasoning with Italian, salt, and pepper.Add the avocados and a tablespoon of pepper, lemon juice, and pesto to the bowl. Set aside the mashed avocados.Place the zucchini noodles on a serving platter, then top with the avocado mixture and salmon.Garnish with cheese. If necessary, add more pesto. Enjoy!

Nutrition:

- ✓ 128 kilocalories
- ✓ 9.9 g fat
- ✓ 9 g total carbohydrates
- ✓ 4 g of protein

84 Cakes with Salmon

Time to Prepare: 15 minutes

Time to cook: 15 minutes

4 servings

Ingredients:
- ✓ half a lemon, zested
- ✓ 6 tbsp of vegetable oil
- ✓ 2 strips cooked and crumbled rasher bacon, bacon fat reserved
- ✓ 2 oz. chopped onion
- ✓ 2 tablespoons grated Parmesan
- ✓ 1 egg
- ✓ 12 teaspoon breadcrumbs
- ✓ 12 cups of mayonnaise
- ✓ 1 potato, baked or boiled, peeled, and fluffed with a fork
- ✓ 2 tsp. Dijon mustard
- ✓ 1 wild salmon tin (14 oz)
- ✓ granulated sugar, 1/2 teaspoon
- ✓ To taste, freshly ground black pepper

Directions:
Preheat 1 tablespoon of reserved bacon fat in a pan over medium heat. Cook for a few minutes or until the onions are translucent. Allow 10 minutes for the onions to cool.Combine mayonnaise, Dijon mustard, lemon zest, cooked onions, bacon, 1/2 teaspoon sugar, and 1 egg in a mixing bowl. Mix thoroughly before adding the potato and

salmon. Form the mixture into 12 patties.In a separate bowl, combine 2 tablespoons of grated parmesan, pepper, and breadcrumbs. Coat the patties one at a time in this mixture.Heat 3 tablespoons of oil in a skillet. Cook the salmon cakes in batches. Cook both sides for 3-4 minutes or until golden. If necessary, add more oil.Place on a serving platter and serve!

Nutrition:

- ✓ 395 kilocalories
- ✓ 32.7 g fat
- ✓ 19 g total carbohydrates
- ✓ Protein content: 7 g

85 Stir-Fry with Chicken and Snap Peas

Time to Prepare: 15 minutes

Time to cook: 10 minutes

4 servings

Ingredients:

- ✓ 14 cups thinly sliced boneless skinless chicken breast
- ✓ 3 tbsp. chopped fresh cilantro
- ✓ 2 tbsp of vegetable oil
- ✓ 2 teaspoons sesame seeds
- ✓ 1 bunch of thinly sliced scallions
- ✓ 2 teaspoons Sriracha sauce
- ✓ 2 minced garlic cloves
- ✓ two tbsp rice vinegar
- ✓ 1 thinly sliced bell pepper
- ✓ 3 tbsp of soy sauce
- ✓ 2 dozen snap peas
- ✓ Season with salt to taste.
- ✓ To taste, freshly ground black pepper

Directions:

In a pan over medium heat, heat the oil. Add the garlic and scallions, thinly sliced. Cook for a minute before adding 2 12 cup snap peas and bell pepper. Cook for 3-4 minutes or until the vegetables are tender.Cook for about 4-5 minutes, or until the chicken is thoroughly cooked.2 teaspoons Sriracha, 2 tablespoons sesame seeds, 3 tablespoons soy sauce, and 2 tablespoons rice vinegar are all good additions. Toss everything together until well combined. Simmer for 2-3 minutes on low heat.Stir in 3 tablespoons of chopped cilantro. If desired, top with additional sesame seeds and cilantro. Enjoy!

Nutrition:

- ✓ 228 kilocalories
- ✓ 11 g fat
- ✓ 11 g total carbohydrates
- ✓ protein (20 g)

86 Chicken Balsamic

Time to Prepare: 15 minutes

Time to cook: 15 minutes

4 servings

Ingredients:

- ✓ 1 pound roasted pumpkin seeds
- ✓ three tbsp olive oil
- ✓ a half-cup of dried cranberries
- ✓ 15-20 trimmed and halved lengthwise Brussels sprouts
- ✓ 1/2 cup non-oil-packed sun-dried tomatoes
- ✓ 1 1/4 lbs. chicken breast, boneless, cut into bite-sized pieces
- ✓ 2 teaspoons honey
- ✓ 1 peeled and diced shallot
- ✓ four tbsp balsamic vinegar

✓ Season with salt to taste.

✓ To taste, pepper

Directions:

In a skillet, heat 2 tablespoons of oil over medium heat. Place the Brussels sprouts cut side down in a bowl. Cook for 4-5 minutes or until seared. Move the Brussels sprouts to the side.Increase the amount of oil in the pan. Add the chicken and shallots. Cook until the chicken is thoroughly cooked, about 4-5 minutes. Season with pepper and salt to taste. Stir in the chicken and flip it over.Drizzle with honey and balsamic vinegar and stir to combine. Cook for a few minutes.Sprinkle the top with 1/2 cup dried cranberries, 1/2 cup sun-dried tomatoes, and 1/2 cup pumpkin seeds. Stir until everything is combined.Serve right away and enjoy!

Nutrition:

✓ 534 kilocalories

✓ 31 g fat

✓ 29 g total carbohydrates

✓ Protein content: 34 g

87 Fried Pineapple Rice

Time to Prepare: 15 minutes

Time to cook: 20 minutes

4 servings

Ingredients:

- ✓ 2 peeled and grated carrots
- ✓ 2 sliced green onions
- ✓ 3 tbsp of soy sauce
- ✓ 1/2 cup diced ham
- ✓ 1 tbsp sesame seed oil
- ✓ 2 cups diced canned/fresh pineapple
- ✓ 1/2 teaspoon ground ginger
- ✓ 3 cups cooked brown rice
- ✓ 1/4 teaspoon ground white pepper
- ✓ 2 tbsp of olive oil
- ✓ 1 frozen cup of peas
- ✓ 2 minced garlic cloves
- ✓ 1 frozen cup of corn
- ✓ 1 diced onion

Directions:

In a mixing bowl, combine 1 tablespoon sesame oil, 3 tablespoons soy sauce, 2 pinches white pepper, and 1/2 teaspoon ginger powder. Mix thoroughly and set aside.Heat the oil in a skillet. Along with the diced onion, add the garlic. Cook for 3-4 minutes, stirring frequently.Next, combine 1/2 cup frozen peas, grated carrots, and 1/2 cup frozen corn in a mixing bowl. Stir for a few minutes or until the vegetables are tender.Next, mix in 2 cups diced pineapple, 12 cups chopped ham, 3 cups cooked brown rice, and sliced green onions. Cook for 2-3 minutes, stirring frequently. Serve!

Nutrition:

- ✓ 252 kilocalories
- ✓ 12.8 g fat
- ✓ 33 g total carbohydrates
- ✓ 3 g of protein

88 Roasted Chicken with Turmeric and Fennel

Time to Prepare: 15 minutes

Time to cook: 45 minutes

6 servings

Ingredients:

- ✓ 3/4 tablespoon turmeric spice
- ✓ 1 thinly sliced lime
- ✓ 1 tablespoon extra virgin olive oil
- ✓ 2 unpeeled and sliced oranges
- ✓ 1/2 cup white wine, dry
- ✓ 6 bone-in, skin-on chicken breasts
- ✓ half a cup of orange juice
- ✓ 1 medium sweet onion
- ✓ 1 lime, squeezed
- ✓ 1 bulb fennel, cored and sliced
- ✓ 2 tbsp of yellow mustard
- ✓ three tbsp brown sugar
- ✓ 1 teaspoon paprika dulce
- ✓ 1 tbsp. garlic powder
- ✓ 1 teaspoon coriander powder
- ✓ Season with salt to taste.
- ✓ To taste, pepper

Directions:

Preheat the oven to 475 degrees Fahrenheit.In a mixing bowl, combine the lime juice, 1/2 cup olive oil, 1/2 cup orange juice, 1/2 cup dry white wine, 3 tablespoons brown sugar, and 2 tablespoons yellow mustard.Transfer half of this spice mixture to the prepared marinade. In another bowl, combine 1 tablespoon garlic powder, 1 teaspoon ground coriander, pepper, salt, 3/4 tablespoon turmeric spice, and 1 teaspoon sweet paprika. Mix until well combined.Pat dry the chicken pieces and season with the remaining spice mix. Combine this chicken with the remaining marinade ingredients in a mixing bowl. Mix.Cover and chill for 1-2 hours before transferring the chicken to a baking pan with the marinade and roasting for 40-45 minutes. Serve immediately!

Nutrition:
- ✓ 559 kilocalories
- ✓ 36.3 g fat
- ✓ 26 g total carbohydrates
- ✓ Protein content: 34 g

89 Salmon Roasted with Potatoes and Romaine

Time to Prepare: 15 minutes

Time to cook: 30 minutes

4 servings

Ingredients:

- ✓ 2 romaine lettuce hearts, cut in half
- ✓ 1 lb. Yukon Gold baby potatoes
- ✓ 14 teaspoons of paprika
- ✓ 14 cup olive oil (distributed)
- ✓ 1 tablespoon melted butter
- ✓ 1 tsp. lemon juice
- ✓ 4 fillets of salmon
- ✓ Season with salt to taste.
- ✓ To taste, freshly ground black pepper

Directions:

Toss the potatoes in a bowl with 2 tablespoons of oil. Place the potatoes on a baking sheet that has been greased. Preheat the oven to 400 degrees Fahrenheit.Cook for 15-20 minutes or until fork-tender and golden.Mix the lemon juice and 2 tablespoons of oil into the romaine hearts. To taste, season with pepper and salt. Set aside.Brush the salmon with melted butter. Sprinkle paprika, pepper, and salt over each fillet.Arrange the salmon, romaine, and potatoes on a baking sheet. Roast for 7-8 minutes.Place on a serving platter and serve!

Nutrition:

- ✓ 611 kilocalories
- ✓ 40 g fat
- ✓ 25 g total carbohydrates
- ✓ 39 grams of protein

90 Soup with Chicken and Gluten-Free Noodles

Time required for preparation: 10 minutes

Cooking Time: 25 minutes

Servings: 4

Ingredients:

- ✓ ¼ cup extra-virgin olive oil
- ✓ 3 celery stalks, sliced 1/4 inch thick
- ✓ 2 medium carrots diced to 1/4-inch
- ✓ 1 tiny onion diced to 1/4-inch size
- ✓ 1 sprig of fresh rosemary
- ✓ 4 cups of chicken stock
- ✓ 8 ounces of gluten-free penne
- ✓ 1 teaspoon salt
- ✓ 1/4 milligram of freshly ground black pepper

- ✓ 2 cups of diced roast chicken
- ✓ 14 cups of freshly chopped flat-leaf parsley

Directions:

In a big saucepan over high heat, heat the oil. The celery, carrots, onion, and rosemary should be sautéed for 5 to 7 minutes or until tender. Bring to a boil the stock, pasta, salt, and pepper. Cook for 8 to 10 minutes at a simmer until the penne is cooked. Remove the rosemary sprig and discard it, then add the chicken and parsley. Turn the heat down to low. Prepare within five minutes and serve.

Nutrition:

- ✓ Calories: 485
- ✓ Total Fat: 18g
- ✓ Total Carbohydrates: 47g
- ✓ Sugar: 4g
- ✓ Fiber: 7g
- ✓ Protein: 33g
- ✓ Sodium: 1423mg

CHAPTER 06: SOME DESSERTS AND SNACK RECIPES

91 Chips made from sweet potatoes

Time to prepare: 20 minutes

2 hours of cooking time

6 servings

Ingredients:

- ✓ 3 tbsp extra virgin olive oil
- ✓ 1 tablespoon sea salt
- ✓ 2 large sweet potatoes, thinly sliced

Directions:

Turn on the oven and set the temperature to 250°F. Place the oven rack in the center. In a large mixing bowl, combine the sweet potato slices and olive oil. Arrange the slices on two baking sheets, one on top of the other, and sprinkle with sea salt. Place the sheets in a preheated oven and bake for about two hours, rotating the pans and flipping the chips after 45 - 60 minutes. Remove the chips from the oven as soon as they are light brown and crisp. Some may be mushy at first, but they will crisp up as they cool. Allow the chips to cool for ten minutes before serving. Serve immediately. After a few hours, the chips will become mushy again.

Nutrition:

- ✓ 43g carbohydrate
- ✓ 2.7g protein
- ✓ 11.1g total fat
- ✓ 268 calories
- ✓ 0.0mg cholesterol
- ✓ 6.5g fiber
- ✓ 483mg sodium

92 Strawberry Chia Ice Pops

Time to Prepare: 5 hours

Time to cook: 0 minutes

6 servings

Ingredients:

- ✓ 2 cups thawed frozen unsweetened strawberries
- ✓ 1 can (15 oz.) coconut milk
- ✓ 1 teaspoon of chia seeds
- ✓ 1 tbsp lemon juice, freshly squeezed
- ✓ a tsp vanilla extract

Directions:

Arrange six ice pop molds or prepare them according to the manufacturer's instructions. In a medium mixing bowl, combine the chia seeds, strawberries, lemon juice, coconut milk, and vanilla extract. Allow the mixture to sit for 5 minutes to allow the chia seeds to thicken slightly. Divide the mixture evenly among the molds. Fill each mold with one ice pop stick. Freeze the pops for about 5 hours or overnight. Serve.

Nutrition:

- ✓ 10g carbohydrate
- ✓ 2.7g protein
- ✓ 17.5g total fat
- ✓ 188 calories
- ✓ 0.0mg cholesterol
- ✓ 3.2g fiber
- ✓ 12mg sodium

93 Cookies with Carob Chips

12 servings

3 cookies per serving

Time to prepare: 10 minutes

Time to cook: 8 minutes

18 minutes to completion

Ingredients

- ✓ 3/4 cup unrefined honey
- ✓ 1 pound almond butter
- ✓ 2 quarts almond flour
- ✓ 2 1/4 cups carob chocolate chips (all-natural carob chips from Chatfield's)
- ✓ 1 teaspoon vanilla extract, pure
- ✓ 1 tsp. baking soda
- ✓ 1 tsp. baking powder
- ✓ or to taste, 1/2 teaspoon sea salt
- ✓ 2 free-range organic eggs
- ✓ 1 tsp. Coconut oil (for greasing)

Directions

Preheat the oven to 375°F. Prepare and grease a baking sheet. Mix the almond butter, honey, eggs, and vanilla extract in a medium bowl. Sift together the baking soda, gluten-free flour mix, baking powder, and salt in a separate bowl salt. Incorporate the butter mixture. Make sure to combine everything thoroughly. Finally, stir in the carob.Chips Using a teaspoon, drop the cookie mixture onto a baking sheet 2 inches apart. Bake, the baking sheet for 8 minutes or until the cookies turn light brown. Allow the cookies to cool for 2 minutes before removing them from the baking sheet.

94 Sandwiches with Almond Butter and Bananas on Gluten-Free Bread

8 servings

1 sandwich = 1 serving

Time to prepare: 15 minutes

15 minutes to prepare

Ingredients

- ✓ 1 tablespoon coconut oil

- ✓ 1 pound almonds
- ✓ 10 drops stevia liquid (or raw honey)
- ✓ 1 teaspoon salt, or to taste
- ✓ 16 gluten-free slicedslices of bread
- ✓ 8 ripe bananas, cut in half lengthwise

Directions

In a food processor, thoroughly combine coconut oil, almond nuts, stevia, and salt until it resembles a butter paste. Allow cooling. Spread 2 tablespoons of almond butter on each pair of gluten-free loaves of bread, then top with banana slices. Serve.

Parfait Citrus Berry

5 servings

1 parfait glass (serving size)

Time to prepare: 10 minutes

10 minutes to prepare

Ingredients

- ✓ 1 cup melted coconut butter

- ✓ 1/2 cup low-fat organic lemon yogurt
- ✓ 1 cup blackberries or blueberries, fresh
- ✓ 1 cup fresh strawberries or raspberries
- ✓ 2 tbsp. unrefined honey
- ✓ 1 cup chopped walnuts or almonds

Directions

Mix honey, lemon yogurt, and coconut butter in a small bowl. Thoroughly. Combine the blackberries and raspberries in a separate bowl. In parfait glasses, layer the berries and coconut butter mixture and top with walnuts on top.

95 Chocolate Cupcakes Without Gluten

12 servings

1 cup of cake per serving

Time to prepare: 10 minutes

Time to cook: 20 minutes

30 minutes to prepare

Ingredients

- ✓ 1 pound almond butter
- ✓ Gluten-Free Self-Rising Flour 130 g
- ✓ Gluten-Free Vanilla Powder 130 g
- ✓ 12 teaspoon carob powder
- ✓ 12 tbsp pure vanilla extract
- ✓ 3 tbsp. unrefined honey
- ✓ 2 free-range organic eggs

Icing:

- ✓ 1 pound almond butter
- ✓ Stevia (100g)

Directions

Preheat the oven to 190°C. Line a standard cupcake tin (12) with paper liners cupcakes). Mix the honey and butter in a medium bowl until fluffy and pale. Include the Blend in the eggs, carob powder, and flour. Bake the mixture in a cupcake tin lined with paper liners for 20 minutes. To make the icing, combine the stevia and butter in a mixing bowl until soft and light. Place the stevia and butter mixture in a piping bag. Place the icing on top of every cupcake

96 Chocolate Garbanzo Bean Cake

12 servings

Time to prepare: 30 minutes

Time to cook: 40 minutes

1 hour 10 minutes to completion

Ingredients

- ✓ 1 1/2 cups semisweet gluten-free chocolate chips
- ✓ 5 tbsp of almond butter
- ✓ 1 can (19 oz.) rinsed and drained garbanzo beans
- ✓ 4 eggs
- ✓ 3/4 cup brown sugar, unrefined
- ✓ a half teaspoon baking powder
- ✓ 1 tbsp cocoa powder, unsweetened
- ✓ 159
- ✓ 1 teaspoon vanilla extract, pure
- ✓ 1 teaspoon of coconut oil

Directions

Preheat the oven to 350° F. (175 degrees C). Grease a 9-inch round cake pan with cooking spray using coconut oil. In a microwave-safe bowl, combine the chocolate chips and almond butter. Cooking in the Microwave for 2 minutes or until completely melted and smooth. In a food processor, combine the beans and eggs and process until smooth. Mix in the sugar, baking powder, melted chocolate mixture,and vanilla extract; blend until smooth and well combined.

Pour the batter into the prepared cake pan. Bake for 40 minutes until a toothpick inserted into the cake comes out clean or only a few crumbs are stuck. Cool for 10-15 minutes in the pan on a wire rack minutes. Turn out onto a serving plate and sprinkle with cocoa powder. Serve.

97 Vanilla Ice Cream with Poached Pears and Chocolate-Mango Sauce

8 servings

1/2 poached pear per serving

Time to prepare: 15 minutes

Time to cook: 16 minutes

31 minutes to completion

Ingredients
- ✓ 1 cup mango nectar (organic)
- ✓ 1 cup white wine, dry
- ✓ 1/2 cup brown sugar, unrefined
- ✓ 4 peeled, halved and cored slightly underripe pears
- ✓ 4 ounces chopped semisweet chocolate
- ✓ 1 cup low-fat, gluten-free vanilla ice cream

Directions

In a large saucepan, combine the pear nectar, white wine, and sugar and boil on medium-high heat. Reduce the heat to medium-low and add the pears. Simmer for 8 minutes, covered, or until Pears are soft. Transfer pear halves to individual plates, cut side up, using a slotted spoon. Increase the heat to medium-high. Boil the poaching liquid for 8 minutes or until it is syrupy and thick, reduced by one-quarter. Remove the pan from the heat. Whisk in the chocolate until it is melted. The sauce is silky. Drizzle warm honey over each pear half and top with 2 tablespoons vanilla ice cream chocolate dipping sauce

98 Baked Almond-Stuffed Apples with Almond Whipped Cream

6 servings

1 stuffed apple per serving

Time to prepare: 20 minutes

Time to cook: 20 minutes

40 minutes to completion

Ingredients

- ✓ six apples

- ✓ 1/2 cup crushed almonds
- ✓ 3 tbsp. unrefined honey
- ✓ 1/2 teaspoon nutmeg
- ✓ a quarter teaspoon of cinnamon
- ✓ 2 small lemons, zest
- ✓ two tbsp almond butter
- ✓ 1 tsp sea salt
- ✓ Whipped Almond Cream:
- ✓ 1 1/2 cups low-fat, gluten-free whipping cream
- ✓ 1 teaspoon almond extract, pure
- ✓ 1/2 teaspoon nutmeg, ground
- ✓ 1 teaspoon cinnamon powder
- ✓ 1 tbsp unrefined honey

Directions

Preheat the oven to 375°F. With a paring knife, remove the apple cores and cut a 1/2-inch slice from the apple base of each apple Place the cored apples in a baking dish and flatten them. Each apple should be filled with almond nuts and crushed.Mix the honey, nutmeg, cinnamon, and lemon zest in a mixing bowl. Add the stuffed apples to a bowl. Combine almond butter and salt in a mixing bowl. 1 teaspoon almond butter on top of each apple mixture. Stuffed apples should be baked for 20-30 minutes. Place the baked apples on serving plates. In a blender or food processor, combine all the whipped cream ingredients and Blend until smooth and creamy. Top each stuffed apple with 2 tablespoons of almond whipped cream.

99 Berry Medley Walnut Parfait with Vanilla Coconut Ice Cream

6 servings

1 parfait glass (serving size)

Time to prepare: 20 minutes

20 minutes to prepare

Ingredients

- ✓ 1 1/2 cups sliced fresh strawberries
- ✓ 1 cup blueberries, fresh
- ✓ 1 cup raspberries, fresh
- ✓ 1 lime, squeezed
- ✓ 1 tbsp unrefined honey
- ✓ 1 cup chopped walnuts
- ✓ Vanilla Coconut Ice Cream
- ✓ 2 cups organic full-fat coconut milk, ice cold
- ✓ 1/2 cup pure honey
- ✓ 1 tsp pure vanilla extract

Directions

To make the Coconut Vanilla Ice Cream, whisk together the coconut milk, honey, and vanilla extract in a food processor Blend on High until smooth and frothy, covered. Fill a container halfway with the liquid. Cover the ice cream bowl and start the ice cream maker to churn it. Transferring to a Freeze in a freezer-safe container; cover and serve. Six parfait glasses should be chilled. In a mixing bowl, combine the berries and drizzle with honey and fresh lime juice. Layer the berries, walnuts, and coconut ice cream in parfait glasses.

BONUS - COOKING TIPS&TRICKS

Scan the code with your mobile phone and download your bonus. Enjoy!

https://bit.ly/Nancy_BONUS

CONCLUSION

Beginning an anti-inflammatory diet might be challenging. There are several regulations to observe, foods to avoid, and recommendations to adhere to.

However, this is what makes it so successful! It helps you eliminate the items that are bad for you and guarantees that you give your body the good things by removing the bad stuff, all in the hopes of minimizing inflammation and harmful health impacts on your body. As a newbie, you might be puzzled about how to begin this diet plan. However, do not let this deter you! The following advice will ensure you get the most out of your anti-inflammatory diet.

Find Someone to Follow the Diet with You.

When it comes time to begin the anti-inflammatory diet, you should evaluate whether you can locate a companion who is prepared to do so with you. Like any diet plan, this can be tiresome and difficult to follow on your own.

It is not easy to adhere to this diet when you observe people around you eating and enjoying whatever they choose while focusing on eating just specific things. And if you were previously an unhealthy person who ate poorly and barely exercised, this will be much more challenging. Having a companion who can collaborate with you and keep you on track will significantly impact you. You may share recipes, discuss difficult situations, and offer one another the necessary support to feel your best.

Find Some Delicious Recipes

When reviewing the anti-inflammatory diet, you will likely find a great deal of information regarding items to avoid.

The list will appear lengthy and intimidating, and you may be at a loss for meal preparation ideas. You may enjoy numerous delicious meals and cuisines while following this diet plan.

But because our brains will be preoccupied with the items we are not permitted to eat, rather than all of the healthy meals we may enjoy, we will lose concentration, worry, and have difficulty.

Finding some decent recipes, such as those contained in this cookbook, will make a significant impact. These might assist you in selecting the scrumptious foods necessary to maintain your health and feel your best.

Take a look at the meal plan and recipes after this book to understand why following this diet plan will be tastier and simpler than you ever dreamed.

Develop Some Inspiration to Help You Stay on Course

Following the anti-inflammatory diet concept might be difficult. If you are not careful and don't have a good level of drive to assist you, it will be much more difficult to get the desired outcomes. Finding a good motivator from the beginning will keep you alive and help you see the desired outcomes, making everything simpler.

Consider why you wish to adhere to this diet plan. Why is it important to see this diet's results and achieve your goals? Interested in weight loss? Do you have widespread discomfort and wish to manage it as much as possible? Are you interested in eliminating some of the health issues that inflammation causes?

You want to keep up with your children and play with them daily, but you're sick of constantly feeling lethargic and weary. Or is there another reason you cannot enjoy things as you like and wish to utilize this as a source of long-term motivation?

Each individual will have their drive, work ethic, and willingness to adhere to the anti-inflammatory diet. And that's all right. It would help if you determined what works best for you and then kept it in a visible location.

Thus, you will continue to take care of yourself and adhere to the anti-inflammatory diet even if things become tough.

Consuming according to the Anti-Inflammatory Diet

The foods this diet allow differing from those permitted on other diet regimens. Because it is vital to emphasize the necessity to avoid inflammatory-causing meals, and it would be best if you consumed a variety of foods that can reduce inflammation in the body.

It would be best if you consumed healthy whole grains, lean meats containing numerous good fats, such as fish, healthy fats, and a variety of fresh produce.

When you can effectively combine all of these factors, you will find it much simpler to realize the health advantages and limit inflammation.

Here are a few tips you may follow to get the most out of your meals while following this diet: Aim for a diet that is rich in diversity.

It will not be fun to follow this diet and consume only a few goods or the same meals each day.

Certainly, this will make things more convenient because you won't need to consider them. However, it won't be long until you become bored. Try to vary the items you consume and add as much color as possible to each dish.

It will prevent boredom and guarantee that your body receives all the nutrition required. It's a healthy game, so enjoy it!

Add fresh ingredients. If you continue consuming junk and processed foods, you will not succeed on this diet. Your meals should be as fresh and nutritious as possible. If you can stick to the outside aisles of the supermarket, you should be fine; avoid fast food and processed items.

These will be loaded with all the toxic nutrients you should avoid, and they will promote inflammation. If you take the time to be on this diet and consume any manufactured food, you will immediately notice the difference. Discourage this as much as possible and eat at home to maintain your health and get the most out of this diet; consume an abundance of fruits. This diet requires you to incorporate more fruits and vegetables into your meals. It will provide your body with the nutrition it requires and assists clear some toxins and free radicals that will create the inflammation you must avoid.

Consider the Elimination Diet

You may want to devote some time to the elimination diet as you work on your anti-inflammatory diet.

It is simple to focus on this concept and guarantee that you eliminate all meals that cause inflammation in the body. Some foods are more likely to produce inflammation but do not cause inflammation in every individual who consumes them.

Sometimes it's okay to consume certain meals, but other times you'll need to avoid them to minimize inflammation. You will perform the elimination diet to determine whether or not this is your problem.

Manufactured by Amazon.ca
Bolton, ON

38466869R00111